Making Doctors

Milo B. Brooks, M.D. and Donna L. Brooks, M.D.

A Century of Lessons on the Practice of Healing

By

Heather Wood Ion

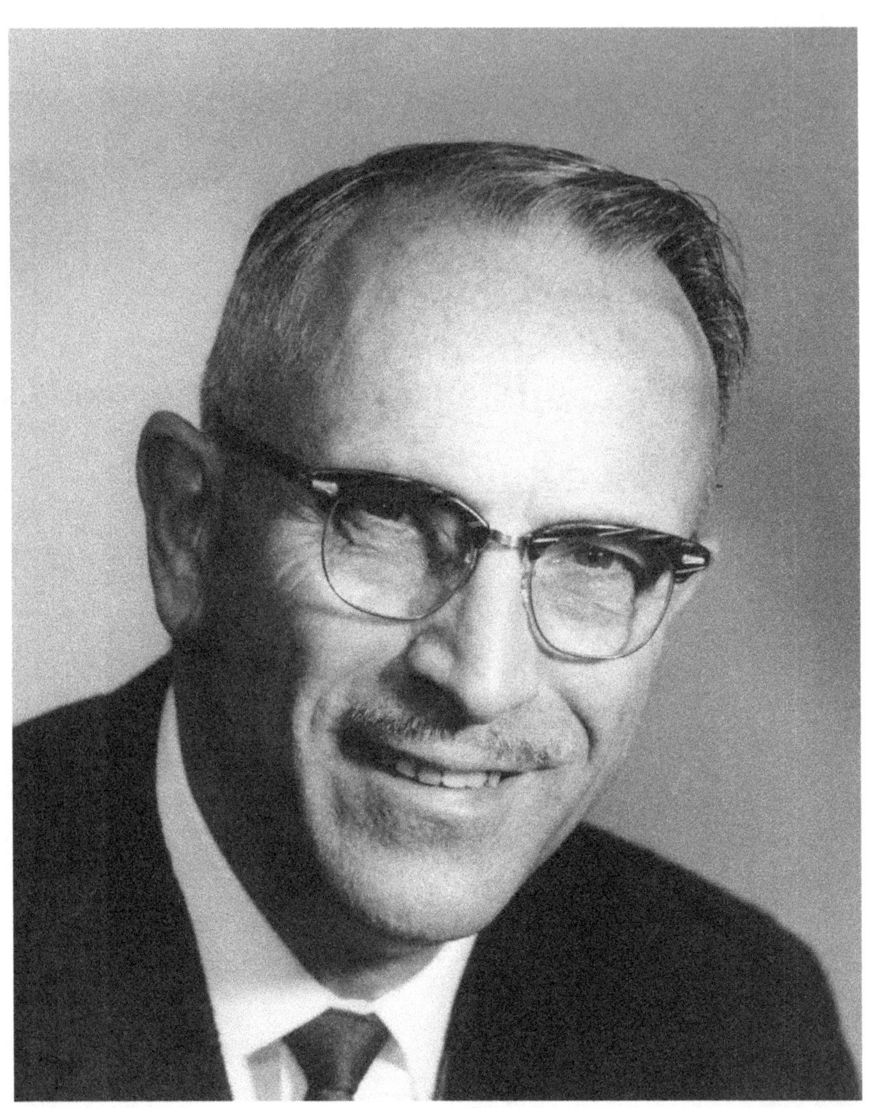

Milo B. Brooks, M.D.

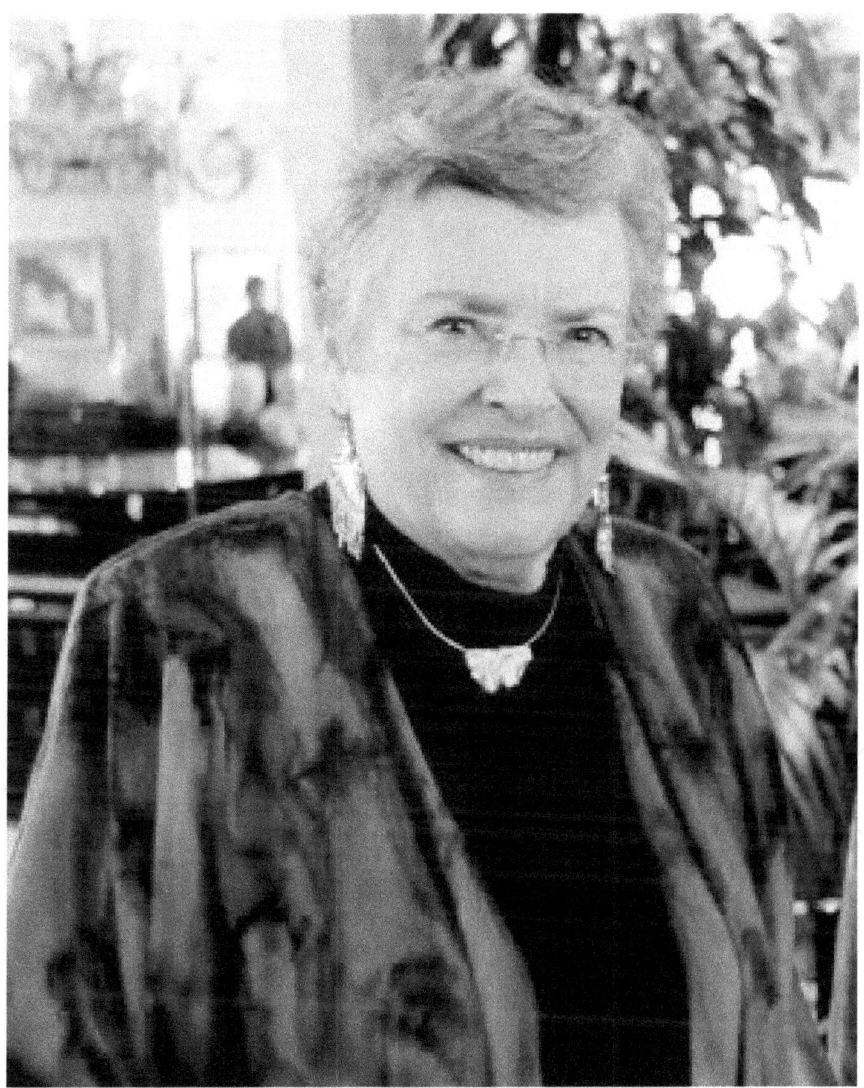

Donna L. Brooks, M.D.

Making Doctors
Milo B. Brooks, M.D. and Donna L. Brooks, M.D.
A Century of Lessons on the Practice of Healing

Copyright © 2013 Heather Wood Ion

All rights reserved. No part of this publication may be reproduced, distributed, or transmitted in any form or by any means, or stored in a database or retrieval system, without the prior written permission of the copyright holder.

10 9 8 7 6 5 4 3 2 1

ISBN 978-0-9898056-0-5

Cover design by Nicholas Ion

Text and layout by Peter Ion

Requests for permission should be directed to
lilascribe@gmail.com

Reprinted by permission of the author:
The poem "Her Hands" by River Malcolm.

Her Hands
Copyright © 1991 by River Malcolm.

DEDICATION

By Donna L. Brooks, M.D.

And on behalf of Milo B. Brooks, M.D.

To our patients, who taught us healing

Contents

ACKNOWLEDGEMENTS

By Donna L. Brooks

Particular thanks to Cathy Conheim for her inspiration for so much of my life and her energetic participation in all our endeavors and projects, including this book.

I wish to pay tribute to the entire Brooks and Crawford families, for their contributions to this story, their closeness over the decades, and to their disciplines in keeping the archive.

Over the years I have received many letters from patients and colleagues expressing their gratitude; for these as constant reminders of what a privilege it is to serve, I am deeply grateful.

Although they have been gone for over twenty years, I thank my parents for their example, for their love, and for their aspirations. My father showed me his love of the practice of medicine.

My thanks to Heather Wood Ion, first and foremost for her friendship, and her patience and support, hard work, encouragement and persistence; without her this book would not have been written.

ACKNOWLEDGEMENTS

By Heather Wood Ion

For encouragement and editing, my thanks to Lenore Ealy. I have long admired the thinking and writing of Richard Gunderman, M.D.; that he has agreed to write the Preface to this book is humbling. I am grateful to him for his inspiring leadership, and for his friendship.

For their editing, layout and commitment to the production of this manuscript, I thank my sons Nicholas and Peter Ion.

Cathy Conheim and Donna Brooks have over the past several years supported my efforts with generosity and kindness and have my deep gratitude and love.

I am profoundly grateful that Donna Brooks has trusted me with this enormous archive, and believe that it is a source of hope as we convey the skills of transformation that we have been shown by our pioneer ancestors.

Preface

Richard Gunderman

It is tempting to suppose that physicians are made through some scientific, technological, or even industrial process. First it is necessary to select students with the appropriate aptitudes, as assayed by a standardized, multiple-choice exam. Then they are conveyed along an assembly line of a curriculum that implants in them the appropriate knowledge and skills, utilizing current pedagogical methodologies. Then assessment techniques verify that the students have learned what they are supposed to know. So long as students of sufficient ability are selected and the curriculum, instructional techniques, and assessment strategies are in order, the inevitable result is a competent physician.

Few things could be further from the truth. The outcomes of medical education and practice are at least as much the product of community, family, and friendship as they are of any formal instructional process. Physicians, and more importantly good physicians, cannot be mass produced, at least not in the same way that we can mass produce automobiles or computers. The machine is an inert thing, entirely the product of its designer's and manufacturer's will, while the physician is a human being, possessed of distinctive life experiences and perspectives, which if not carefully tended, make it impossible for greatness to take root and blossom forth.

The journals of medical education and practice are filled with "scientific" studies, driven by data, statistical techniques, and focused on refuting the null hypothesis. This may work reasonably well when it comes to studying the growth or inhibition of bacterial colonies, but it simply will not do as our path to understanding medical excellence. To account for genuine excellence, we must look beyond the merely quantitative and objective to the qualitative and the subjective. The greatness of the physician is rooted in subjectivity, the ability to understand patients (and self) as knowing, feeling subjects afflicted with illnesses, not diseases that happen to be contained in human husks.

Herein lies the genius of this book. It does not regale us with data. Instead, it tells stories, the stories of remarkable physicians. Where did they come from? What events and experiences shaped their path? What did they at the time think they were doing, and what did they subsequently discover to be the deeper meaning of their life and work? By experiencing vicariously the narrative of a medical life, we are granted the opportunity to peer more deeply into the true wellsprings of medical excellence. In this respect students of medicine–who should read this book–owe a deep debt of gratitude to both the subjects of this book and their chronicler, who remind us what such excellence is really all about.

Richard Gunderman, M.D., Ph.D.

Indiana University

Commentary by Erving Polster

This book tells the story of old-fashioned Americana evolving into exceptional medical accomplishment. It portrays the lives of a father and daughter, Milo and Donna Brooks, who are the culmination of generations of prairie people. While progressing from unschooled and dirt-poor ingenuity into a world of technology, they retained the old simplicity; looking at whatever needs to be done, squarely and without complaint. When they moved into the urban world of complex professional responsibilities, they left the family's primitive environment. But the lessons never left them. As the author writes about this background, "Those who came from farming roots made their lives and our nation by 'just looking beyond'."

Donna and Milo, did, indeed, look beyond their heritage of an earth-bound self-sufficiency, always mindful of the contrasting credo; that people need people. The book imprints the reader with this potent message by making the human dimension colorful and practical. While Milo and Donna were crossovers into the culture of honored physicians, their patients were always more than a technical challenge. First they were people; when that was settled, they could become patients. This book is a testament to a humane life force that percolates underneath all the complexity of our educational advances. Cheers, therefore, for a father and a daughter taking this heritage a step forward, showing us how to carry simple values into distinguished careers.

Erving Polster, Ph.D.

Founder, The Gestalt Training Center, San Diego

Health of the Public from 1900 to 1930

Life Expectancy	Males	Females
1900	46.3	48.3 years

Maternal Mortality 700 deaths per 100,000 births

1900 5% of women gave birth in hospital

Less than half of all births were attended by a physician

1900 On average 10% of children born died before their first birthday

1 out of 5 children died before the age of five

In some US cities, 30% of children died in the first year

1900 Officials estimated 15% of the population was infected by syphilis

1900 Leading Causes of Death

1. Pneumonia and Influenza
2. Tuberculosis
3. Diarrhea and enteritis
4. Heart disease
5. Stroke
6. Nephritic (Kidney) Diseases
7. Accidents
8. Cancer
9. Senility
10. Diphtheria

1903 The American Medical Association adopted the Principles of Medical Ethics due to the issues of venereal disease, confidentiality, and public responsibility.

Advances in medicine over the period

1880 Pasteur established the streptococcal cause of puerperal fever, but the germ basis of disease was slow to be accepted

1890-1910 Isolation was the treatment for infectious diseases

Morphine was the only opiate available

Physicians were not college educated and were trained by apprenticeship

1894 First C-Section performed in Boston

1900 Introduction of water/sand filtration of public water

1908 First Regulation of milk pasteurization in Chicago

1910 Introduction of antiseptic surgery

1921 30% of women gave birth in hospitals

1920-1930 Infant mortality increased due to excessive interventions by physicians (CDC)

1925 Onward: Sewage treatment plants introduced in the US.

1974 First Clean Water Act in the United States

Sources: CDC, MMWR, April 02, 1999/48 (12);243-248 Achievements in Public Health 1900-1999

Leavitt, Judith Walzer, and Numbers, Ronald L.; Sickness & Health in America, Third Edition, University of Wisconsin Press, 1997

Explanation of Format

Making Doctors celebrates the art of healing through the stories of a father and daughter. Both achieved excellence in their fields, and both exemplify the sacred trust inherent in the profession of medicine.

Based on a remarkable archive of memoirs, letters, photographs, interviews and family newsletters, the story takes us from the harsh lives of homesteaders in North Dakota to pioneering innovations in modern medicine. We share the adventures of the Brooks family from prairie fires to heart-wrenching tragedies, and throughout it all we are engaged in the growth of character as a fundamental necessity to the practice of medicine. This is an intimate chronicle of importance for times in which we take the impact of technology for granted and yet, we often forget that it is the humanity we share which heals and gives us hope.

Making Doctors challenges us to remember the debt we owe to the homesteading tradition, to explore the critical questions of whether we are worthy of trust, of what kind of legacy we create in our lives through our relationships with others, and whether we do all that we can to be of service.

Since much of this text comes directly from memoirs, letters and interviews, all those voices are in italics, without changes in grammar etc., while the narrative is in plain text.

Chapter I

The Horses Were Scared of Trees

There were very few buffalo left on the prairie but it was still possible in the summer months to gather buffalo chips to supplement the limited supply of coal. One lone bull did remain and mingle with the neighbors' cattle across the lake. His rare visits to us were occasions to find me under the bed upstairs. One time he did butt his head against the house and make it shake and me tremble.

Milo Brooks became Professor of Pediatrics at UCLA, USC and Loma Linda University, and in reflecting on his success he attributed much to the ways he was shaped by his early, rugged, life. He wrote detailed memoirs richly describing the adventures of his childhood. He was born, the fifth of ten children, in 1898 on the farm in Nashua, Iowa, which had been the 1867 homestead of his grandfather.

How did he do it? How did he make the journey from sod house to professorships in Pediatrics? How did he reflect on the transformation of the medicine he first practiced, prior to antibiotics, to the sophistication of the technologies we today take for granted? What makes a great and innovative healer? He, and his daughter Donna Brooks, who followed in her father's footsteps as a physician, have a legacy to share. It is not only a story in the history of medicine, but a tale of the transformation of American lives and attitudes. It is a story that begins on the cold plains of North Dakota.

Dad decided to homestead a farm in North Dakota in 1901, at thirty-seven years of age, after sixteen years of marriage. A tar paper shack 16 by 24 feet with sod walls and dug into the ground three

> *feet, with a cast iron coal burning cook stove for heat and homemade furniture, mother had her first home of her own. There was as yet no well, and water was hauled in barrels from the lake a half mile away or from melted snow. In either case it had to be boiled for drinking. Clothes were freeze dried, then hung inside for final drying. Family baths were in a galvanized iron tub with care to save water.*
> *By next July, the seventh child, my sister Julia, was born.*

All of the children were born at home, sometimes with a doctor in attendance. Their births were recorded in the family Bible, as well as one daughter's death—Lulu, who died at six months of age of pneumonia. As was typical at the time, the parents of this brood had little formal education but were driven to both educate themselves and see that all of the children were educated, despite long absences from formal schooling for planting and harvest, and for hard times. Ellsworth Elmer Brooks and Melvina Azilda Brunais Brooks epitomized the pioneer virtues of their fellow homesteaders. They raised all of their children to work hard and solve whatever challenges they faced. Sometimes the whole family moved from farm to town for the sake of schooling, and then back to the farm to maintain cash flow.

Milo's oldest brother Maurice describes the conditions:

> *When we moved to North Dakota on March 1, 1901, it was about the middle of the school year, and I didn't attend school for a year or two, except for part time, and none of us were able to attend school regularly because there was none nearby, and usually schools were open only during the summer because of the severe winters. I had to help with the farm work, hand digging a well and building both a barn and house in that order. At first we all lived in a one-room shack built of one inch lumber and covered with tar paper held in place by strips*

> *of lath, on both the roof and sides, and it was heated with a sizeable kitchen stove with coal fire, as this was prairie country and we could hardly find enough wood for kindling.*
>
> *It might seem impossible that all eight of us could crowd into such a space of about sixteen by twenty-four feet, but we managed pretty well with the back-house outside.*

Maurice was fourteen at this time, driving the breaking plows into the virgin prairie with a five horse team. He finished seventh grade, and then in 1905 took a first year of high school.

> *In the spring of 1906 the Towner County Superintendent of Schools insisted that I take the Teacher's Examination, and when I passed he assigned me to a summer school in the country about ten miles south-west of our home where some problem boys in the school had frightened a lady teacher into resigning. I rode horseback over and back there daily.*
>
> *In the fall of 1906 we all came back to Nashua, Iowa with Grandma Brooks again, leaving Mom and Dad on the North Dakota farm until they could get everything closed out there and come back to Iowa with all of us where we could attend a good school. I finished the last three years of High School there graduating in 1909, and all the other children continued in school there and finished high school there.*

Milo would later, at age fifteen, also become a substitute teacher, and it is an indication of the discipline of the parents that these teenage boys were put in responsible positions so young. But in 1901, Milo was still a toddler when one of the most dramatic events of his childhood took place.

> *The prairie was flat and treeless. A six-foot high willow bush by the lake was the only tree I knew until, when I was eight, we drove our wagons for a vacation in the Turtle Mountains near Rollo. The Langdon Trail crossed a corner of our farm and Indian tribes of the Sioux nation followed this route from Canada. ... Fall came and after the harvest, the prairie fire. A long Black cloud east of us extended from horizon to horizon and kept coming. Dad and Maurice harnessed all the horses to plows and started to plow firebreak furrows around our buildings. Dad got on the barn roof with a water bucket and mop, and someone likewise was on the house. Maurice chased all the livestock into the barn and hitched one team, Rock and Lightfoot, to the water tank wagon to spray water inside and outside the firebreak. Each of us had a bucket and mop or wet towel of some sort and prepared for the battle. [Milo was three years old.] The flames leaped fifteen feet high as they raced faster than a horse could run. Maurice and the team were caught outside the firebreak and by aiming the hose on the horses while he pumped, he was able to come out with only slightly singed horses. We were all busy swatting out little fires that kept starting everywhere in the yard. Suddenly it was over and the flames raced on to the lake where they parted and spared our neighbor's home across the lake. No buildings were burned nor person or animals more than singed in our immediate area. The flat prairie was black as far as one could see in any direction.*

In comparison with child-rearing a century later, it is difficult to conceive of a group of children being called upon to help their parents and grandmother in such an emergency today, yet clearly the Brooks children were trusted to help and know what to do. Milo often recounts his own mischief, but the farm required that everyone contribute as soon as they were able.

Milo persuaded his mother to let him go off to school at age four with the four elder children, when Maurice was the temporary teacher. At recess older children would set snares for the gophers, trying to collect the bounty of two cents per gopher tail. Milo was once late returning from recess and the attempt to catch a gopher:

> *On entering school late [I] was sternly met by the teacher—my brother Maurice—who felt compelled to be more strict with his brothers and sisters than with others. His punishment was having me sit at one of the school's double desks between two girls. I enjoyed it.*
>
> *One other time I was scolded for tracing lice travels on my notebook paper. The girl in front of me had long braids that hung on my desk. An occasional louse would leave the braids for a stroll across my note paper. (We all had lice at Balton School.) It was fun following the louse travels with my pencil. But it amused the two boys behind me and they laughed.*

Milo's sense of fun helped him become an effective pediatrician, and he would later write of making toys and playground equipment for his children's school. The reader of the diaries is frequently astounded by both the responsibility and the competence required of the children.

Here is Milo describing what he was dealing with at age 10:

> *We raised Percheron and Belgian draft horses for sale and did the farm work with brood mares and colts. Those huge colts that we had raised as pets when they were little now had lots of life and power and often ran away.*
>
> *Once I had four of the big one ton colts hitched to a disk harrow. This is a big cultivating tool about sixteen feet wide and equipped with a disk every six inches. It would cut the rough plowed field into*

tillable soil. As we were stopped to rest one of the colts kicked over his trace in fighting flies. It frightened him and I was not able to unfasten the trace in the narrow dangerous space between the horses and the disk. I went to his head and tried to calm him and possibly unfasten the trace from that end. However, I was not able to do that and all four horses were excited and began rearing up on the hind legs and coming toward me. I was able to get away and grab for the reins on the machine but missed. Now they were running with the disk harrow so fast that it jumped thirty feet between times it hit the ground. I ran behind crying for fear my lovely horses would get badly hurt.

Before long the two center horses fell and the sharp disks were pulled over them. I rapidly unfastened the traces but got only one horse loose and the other three got up and ran until they pulled in opposite directions and had to stop. I got one more horse loose and then another. The last horse still dragged the disk until I could run him into a hay stack.

I was so relieved when I got them all unharnessed and in the barn to find none of them had deep cuts. But the harnesses were in shreds and four new harnesses would cost over $200. I was in the harness shop repairing when Dad came in. He said nothing but sat down to help and the next day we had the harnesses repaired and the four colts working in the field again .

Here, at ten, the future healer is obvious: he is concerned for injury to the animals in his care, he does the very best he can to get them to safety, and then he repairs what is broken. I picture him sitting in the barn: he was small for his age, so the broken harness for a four horse team would have been heavy and cumbersome. All the work would have to be done by hand, and we must imagine that Milo had learned the skills by observing others, but at least in this story, he sets about his task alone, without being daunted.

Three years earlier, when he was seven years old, Milo took a small boy's delight in watching the building of the railroad in North Dakota. He recounts his fascination with the pile drivers and conveyor belts and the crews hammering the rails with spikes into the ties.

> *It was a lot of fun and excitement to see this modern system of laying railroad continuously. The railroad switching yards were laid just north of our house and a string of four elevators were eventually built along that street. Our excitement came in the fall when the trains would come along to pick up the grain that had been stored in the elevators. They would switch the cars off onto the sidings and we children would grab onto a freight car that had been flying switch and ride it to the end. How we ever managed not to fall and get cut to pieces is a wonder.*

Thinking about all these adventures, we imagine Milo's mother, a French-speaking girl from northern New York state who could not have imagined the rigor of life on the prairies of Iowa and North Dakota, let alone that she would eventually have ten children to raise. Milo reflects on his mother's life:

> *It must have been in the fall of 1906 or 1907 when I was in school in the basement chasing little lizards; Mother was getting pretty fed up with North Dakota. It had been a very hard life on her, having lost her eighth child Lulu, having run a hotel, and now Maurice and Delia and Rena [the three eldest children] and Grandma Brooks had gone back to Nashua, Iowa so that they could go to high school. Mother was staying in Rock Lake [North Dakota] with us younger children. We were constantly getting into mischief of all kinds. Mother had decided*

that she had had enough of that and she wanted to civilize her Indians and move to Iowa.

To make this journey, the family had first to ride in the caboose of a freight train to Minneapolis, the children terrifying both the conductor and their mother most of the way. They missed the connection and had to spend twenty-three hours in the depot before finally catching the passenger train on to Nashua. Milo makes no comment on his mother's mood by the time she settled her brood safely into a little house near the family farm. Months later, Mr. Brooks joined the family:

> *Dad came when snow closed in on Rock Lake and brought the horses down in a freight car. They were frightened of trees, having never seen one. I remember how they would shy and be frightened to go in the shade of a tree.*

Milo recalls with particular fondness the small pony, Trixie, which delighted all the children for most of her life.

> *She was privileged to have the freedom of the farm yard with its delicious green lawn, and was not tied up or fenced in. She did like to go to get the cows for evening milking. Often they grazed on the south eighty acres nearly a mile away. I rode her without halter, bridle or saddle and my toes could touch the ground. She loved to herd the cattle and, without any guidance from me, would not let one get behind. The problem was to slow her so as not to worry the milk cows. Later she learned to drive the entire herd of horses. She loved to lord it over the big 2000 pound horses with her little three hundred and fifty pound body. When they challenged her she would stand on her hind feet and cuff them with her front hooves. ...*
>
> *One time in the spring when the ground, which was sometimes frozen six feet deep began to thaw*

and make spongy and muddy roads, my brother Walter got the croup. His cough sounded awful. Mother called Dr. Sutton on the farmers' telephone line. He said "Send someone down and I'll send out some cough medicine." I thought it was urgent. Trixie was frisky and I let her run the two and a half miles and tied her to the hitching post at the doctor's office. He said, "How did you get here? I just hung up the phone."

I tried to slow her going home but she wanted to run. Going down the first hill, I had managed to slow her as there was deep mud at the bottom of the hill. As we neared the mud and I relaxed the reins she accelerated full speed to land knee deep in sticky mud. I slid forward over her ears and head first up to my eyes in the mud. She clambered over me, but I held onto the reins and also grabbed her bushy tail as she went on. I held her long enough to make sure the cough medicine was still in my pocket and to remount. This time I was not angry but rather proud of her speed and spirit and she earned a good rubbing down. The cough syrup seemed to help Walter's cough remarkably well too.

Among the nine surviving children, there must have been many bouts of illness and injury on the farm, but few are mentioned in the diaries. In the early years the family identified as Christian Scientists, which may account for the silence about such things. However, there is at least one dramatic exception:

Whenever I mentioned writing the story of my teenage years, people smile, perhaps feeling that if all were told it might be a luscious story. However it is probably more like most people's lives, interesting and enjoyed but filled with anxieties and fears.

We should start at the age of nine when we had just returned to Iowa from North Dakota and were living in the town of Nashua where I was in the third grade in school. I played with a neighbor boy we shall call Charles who was a freshman in high school. I enjoyed playing marbles with him because I could sometimes win and he would play for fun and not always for keeps and win all my marbles.

He confided his secret episodes with a widow who lived on the edge of town. I was intrigued by his stories, especially as he suggested I might sometime go with him. A short time later he had to interrupt the game of marbles to go behind the barn for urinary relief. The sight I saw of blood and pus and screaming pain was frightening. I had been raised on a farm and knew a lot about sex and of gonorrhea that we called 'clap'. Charles was ill and confined to his home the next few days. A few days later I was told that he had died of pneumonia. Years later in medical college I was to learn of the serious and often rapidly fatal results of gonorrheal pneumonia.

Once again, the dramatic contrast between a childhood today and Milo Brooks' childhood is startling. The skills of the healer, of acute and profound observation, of attending to the whole and not merely a part of the problem, and of taking responsibility for finding a practical solution were developed and reinforced constantly by the value given each individual's ability to work.

Milo wrote "At ten years of age I was greatly thrilled to be allowed to take a man's place in the field." This was not 'child labor' but an acknowledgement of his ability to contribute to the family.

The summer of 1913 was particularly memorable when our round barn was built and I was fascinated, being fifteen years of age, with the details of construction and showed many people who came from a distance to see the curiosity of a round

> *barn. It was 60 feet in diameter and 62 feet high to the center peak. A sixteen foot diameter silo was in the center. Cattle space was in the first story with a concrete floor above to house the horses. On the first floor about half of the area was a stock corral that would hold about 60 loose cattle. The other half had stanchions for about 20 milk cows. On the second floor were stalls for about 30 horses with slightly over a quarter of the area reserved for a drive through and the granary space for wheat and oats.*
>
> *Above under a hip roof was a huge hay loft. Hundreds of visitors came to see the construction and to view the barn in the next year or two and I became an informed tour guide. I could still draw plans to scale of most of the construction. Total cost was about $5000 which was a lot for a poor farmer with a huge family and it proved too much.*

Round barns became popular throughout the Midwest in the first decades of the twentieth century. Raising a barn was one of the family's many traditional skills in which they took great pride.

> *Grandfather was a barn raiser. He cut the heavy timber beams and the mortise and tenons and had them all laid out. When all the neighbors came for the raising, he was ready to fit the tenons in the mortises and drive the wooden pins home. It was a feat of which my father was proud of his father, and was just old enough to remember the raising of our barn. It was always a social occasion with a feast enjoyed by all. Grandpa was the one to shout "heave Ho" as everyone pushed to raise a side.*

The building of the Round Barn was one project that Milo was able to document with photography, and he talked about it with pride throughout his life. Not only would Milo work his way through medical school using these carpentry and mechanical skills, but they would lead him as a pediatrician to establish and direct the Child Amputee Prosthetics Project in California.

In addition to the shared work of major projects, such as barn raisings, which brought the community together, the church and Sunday school were the focus of social life for the family. Like his older brothers and sisters, Milo taught Sunday school and led various youth groups throughout his teenage years.

At first there were only visiting preachers of various denominations Baptists, Methodists, Seventh Day Adventists and Dunkards. In Iowa the family first attended the Little Brown Church (of the hymn) which was Congregationalist, but when the Baptist Church became established, the family joined that. The sermons were robust, often with reference to Harry Emerson Fosdick. Milo's mother had always sung hymns as lullabies, and emphasized repeatedly the need to lead a life of high moral tone.

The tasks on the farm, and especially major projects such as the barn raising, brought Milo and his father together.

> *Dad and I visited a lot doing chores and some in the fields. He was generally quiet and of few words. He talked a lot about his father and his mechanical skills, but Dad himself was most capable. He often said "A man could do almost anything if he had the tools and knew how." There seemed to be nothing on the farm he could not build or repair, and he taught me.*

It is hard to imagine today how grim the responsibilities on the farm could be for the young man. Milo describes the final day of his favorite horse Mollie:

> *One sunny winter day she was lying on a small knoll in the barnyard with her feet higher than her body and was unable to get up on her feet. In this helpless position, the half-grown hogs started eating her and had her intestines strung across the*

yard when I heard her whinny and came to rescue her and chased the hogs away. Dad was away and it was my job to go get the shotgun. I can never forget the look of disbelief she gave me when she saw, and I believe realized, what I was doing.

That was not all of the hard part. The cold night was coming on and she would soon be frozen and we needed her pelt. I was 17 but not too old to cry and sob with every cut as I removed the pelt. It made a warm robe used in the buggy or cutter for many years.

Milo would retain the attitude that he could do almost anything with the right tools and the right skills, and he applied that attitude throughout his life. Nevertheless, Milo began to look for opportunities outside of the unrelenting work of farming. Maurice Brooks had left to study accounting, and Milo would also eventually leave the farm.

Dependence on the weather made farming unstable, even the impact of a cloud of volcanic dust from an eruption in Mexico caused a crop failure in Iowa.

1915 was also a memorable year because it was cold and rainy all summer and there was absolutely no corn to husk and put in the barn. We had a silo in our new round barn and we put as much as we could of our crop in our silo for silage. There was not one single ear of corn ripe enough to husk for grain.

In the winter of 1916 I attended Ames short course for farm boys taking a course in animal husbandry, but after the disaster of 1915 and also a poor crop in 1916 and 1917, I was ready to leave the farm. The war was on in Europe and I was anxious to get activated.

Childhood was over, Milo was ready for adulthood. The next decade would be no less filled with adventures and challenges. The difference now would be that he would both seek and choose his adventures himself. Homesteading had been his grandparents' and father's choice, now Milo sought to find a new path.

Chapter II

Something Positive To DO

The crop failures, and the use of the money from the sale of his hogs to pay the mortgage on the farm rather than his college fees, disheartened Milo about staying on the land. Further, it was discouraging to see the other young men volunteering for war, while he remained responsible for the running of the farm. In August of 1918, Milo joined his friends Stanley Thomas and Sid Gordon, at the International Congress of the Baptist Young People's Union and listened to the preachers John Mott and E. Stanley Jones.

> *The call to be a medical missionary sounded more interesting and romantic than continuing to raise crop failures and go deeper in debt. I hadn't thought much about medicine, but Stanley Thomas was very positive about his plans. Anyway, it sounded better than a missionary preacher: Something positive to do rather than just something to say.*

The Student Army Training Corps provided the opportunity to volunteer and start college with full credit. Stanley and Milo volunteered and signed up for Pre-Med courses at the State University of Iowa. Milo caught influenza in the great pandemic and was ill for a month. It was his first and longest experience of illness. Basic training for the army was even more educational than Milo anticipated:

> *I was a bed wetter to the age of ten. I was very ashamed and worked hard to overcome the problem. I was not unduly scolded or ridiculed but seemed to sleep hard as I worked on the farm. The bed wetting was solved with an alarm clock and a pot under the bed.*

All was well in the army as the latrine, consisting of two parallel ditches six feet deep and two feet wide, was located directly behind the barracks. Two trips a night was no problem. One night past midnight I was awakened by noise from the engineers' barracks nearby where noise was frequent. I headed for the latrine but was grabbed by two guards and ushered back into our barracks.

The noise was from short-arm inspection and the inspectors were now in our barracks. I had no knowledge that a favorite trick of gonorrhea patients was to flush the urethra before inspection. The inspectors found a drop of urine. (I could have given a quart.) He said, "Take him to the Syph Squad." Those with suspected or actual venereal disease were housed in isolation barracks. Inmates were treated exactly like those in the Guard House where I had served as a guard. The bunks were widely spaced and everyone kept to himself with his bunk and belongings. After everyone else had eaten we were marched at attention under guard to the mess hall where the kitchen police served us at arm's length. After each meal we were marched back across the parade ground to our barracks. Soldiers on the parade ground scattered and gave us a wide berth, saying "Here comes the Syph Squad." I had often wondered how the lepers of Biblical times felt going about shouting 'Unclean".

The war ended while Milo was in Basic Training.

On December 19, 1918 we were discharged in time to go home for Christmas. We had a third of a year of college credits in Premed and acceptance to continue with GI credit for free tuition and $1 per day for participation in R.O.T.C.

Stanley Thomas and I were eager to go back. We each got restaurant jobs to pay for our meals

> *with three hours a day work and I added an evening janitor job in the Liberal Arts Building for 25 cents an hour, which paid my room and some money for incidentals. Stanley and his cousin Sid Gordon had been making good money raising onions and potatoes in vacant lots in Osage. We had both been active in the Iowa City Baptist Church and the Sunday School where I had inherited a class of 3rd and 4th grade boys. Every five minute block of time was cherished and allocated.*

Milo describes these first two years of college as busy and happy. The Baptist Young People's Union remained his social anchor, but every waking hour was taken up by work to support his studies, and work back on the farm to help the family. As he was introduced to foreign students, Milo's own horizons were expanding. Some of these friendships would last his entire life. In the summer of 1920 Milo's father sold the farm and moved to Charles City, where he worked in the Hart Parr tractor factory. Milo no longer was torn, now he could focus all his energies on his studies.

> *At the College of Medicine in 1920 all applicants with proper required subjects in two years of college and a grade above C were accepted. The weeding out came in the Freshman year of Medicine, of the one hundred and twenty of us starting, thirty graduated four years later. Most were dropped in the first year.*

Stanley and Milo were working hard to earn cash in their onion and potato business, so they had to come up with a way of dealing with the lectures necessary for their study.

> *Stanley could take shorthand notes and could type. Our professors were blackboard artists and I had to learn to draw, in colors. I also took such notes as I could. In the rapid-fire lectures, strange medical terms were not defined or spelled, so with*

the greatest of ease one could wonder what the man was talking about.

Our plan to meet this was to preview the next assigned lecture in the text and be somewhat familiar with the many new words and their meanings. Then after each lecture and the telegrams (for the produce business) answered, we sat together with me on the text and notes and Stanley on the typewriter. Spaces were left for the drawings that I filled in later. I got the carbon copy and an almost verbatim copy of the lecture with drawings and notations where the lecture differed from the text, which it often did. Each day we reviewed the previous day's lectures, typed up the current day's lectures and previewed the text for the next day's work. There was nothing difficult about this unless you once got behind, but Oh! How voluminous, and we worked long into the night.

This discipline resulted in superb exam scores, with Stanley and Milo being rated 3rd and 4th in the class of 120. But their good fortune vanished when the produce prices fell and their carefully stored potatoes had to be hauled away for fertilizer. Stanley fled, his cousin Sid stayed and paid off the debts over the next ten years. Milo got a teaching job for $120 a month for the winter and in the summer of 1921 worked hard to try to save the farm of a friend. Once more the crop failed, and again, Milo did the back breaking work of running the farm, milking the cows, cleaning stables, taking the children of his friend back and forth to school five and a-half miles each way through the winter. By the autumn of 1923 the bank took the farm.

Milo had now postponed continuing college for two years and still had no money saved, but he was determined to finish his education. At Des Moines University, Milo wanted to take 24 semester hours to make up for lost time. The Dean agreed that he could try to do 21 but must drop any course in which he made less than a B.

> *I paid my $7 down on tuition and took a job as a campus caretaker in charge of trimming lawn and shrubs with a team of horses in an on-campus barn to take care of. This was to pay the rest of my tuition and room in the men's dorm, Johnson Hall. I loved that old team of horses and could study some while riding the lawn mower. For food, the restaurant across the street gave me three meals for three hours work, 5:00 am to 8: 00 am. I opened up, prepared, and served the breakfasts.*
>
> *Budgeting of time was most important and I still was able to manage some janitor work for cash income. The twenty-one credit hours was easier than medical college but the Educational Psychology was a challenge. The professor assigned me to read, outline, and pass an exam on a complete textbook each week. I still have my first assigned text—Tishner's Educational Psychology. He gave me a B+ in the course. I had learned to like a challenge.*

In the second semester, Milo took a job which reflects the young man he was and the physician he would become. He became the caregiver for Professor Fulcher who taught Physics and Bible studies. The professor had a progressive paralytic disease (a demyelinizing process of the spinal motor nerves) so Milo began by reading his lectures for him, doing the driving, and finally providing the personal care at home which his wife could not provide. Milo earned board and room and a small stipend, but "The most stimulating experience was the many conversations we had on his notebook. His hearing and all sensory functions were intact so I did not have to write."

> *Professor Fulcher became weaker and weaker and as school ended in the spring required my full time attention night and day. He had lost weight and had to be turned in bed several times a night. I slept on a cot near him and the ability I had learned to awaken and then go back to sleep at the drop of an*

> *eyelid became valuable. We continued with the Sunday school and church all summer.*

The urgent need to earn enough to save for a return to college prompted Milo to apply to several high schools for a position as an athletic coach as well as manual training and science teacher: Coon Rapids, Iowa hired him for the autumn term. He had difficulty leaving Professor Fulcher and after only a week away was called to return for the Professor's funeral. The complete involvement of the caregiver in all aspects of the patient's life was a lesson Milo would never forget, and would later prompt him always to inform the family quickly and clearly of whatever was happening with his patient.

> *I was very careful to save every single dollar I could in this one year and was anxious to be back in medical college the next fall. That summer, 1925, I worked in the forge shop of the Hart Parr factory of Charles City, Iowa. My parents lived in a large house just a few blocks from the factory, and staying at home saved board and room and I saved some more money.*

By the fall of 1925, Milo was again enrolled in medicine in Iowa City.

> *It was stupid to be working such long hours and studying medicine and trying out for football. ... There wasn't much danger of me not doing my medical studying, the subjects were fascinating and I was charged with the responsibility of keeping my grades in the upper third of the class or be dropped. During the winter as I needed cash income—at twenty-five cents per hour—I found that I could work the eight hour shift, midnight to eight in the morning in the bakery without interfering with classes. The year was pleasant and I did finish well in the upper third. It seemed I was always pushing myself to take in one more interesting experience, enjoying it to*

the fullest and making that experience part of me.

The final sentence in the paragraph summarizes Milo's attitudes and choices as he worked constantly toward his goal.

Let us pause here and think of the state of medicine and medical education in 1925. Infectious diseases were the constant fear, the influenza pandemic of 1918 revealed just how little doctors could do against such diseases. There were as yet no antibiotics, the *materia medica* was much as it had been for centuries, WWI had taught physicians a great deal about orthopedics, but for the public scourges of tuberculosis and venereal disease little could be done. Medical education had lately changed from the apprenticeship system to the lecture system based in a hospital, and schools were striving to establish shared standards of knowledge and skill. Doctors practiced in the home and from home, patients went to the hospital only as a last resort, or when isolation of the patient was deemed necessary.

Another crop failure meant that Milo returned to school without any money.

> *The hospital was trying to find a student to work twelve hours a night, seven to seven, six days a week, as a floor orderly on men's medical where there were many serious and terminal cases.*
> *I offered to take it every other night and share it with another student. The personnel director refused the split so in desperation I took the job.*
>
> *This sophomore year was full of lab courses and the schedule, eight to five daily to Saturday noon, had every hour filled except one hour on Wednesday. The job solved my room problem; the nurses let me use one corner of the nursing station for my books and studying. My experience in using every possible minute between calls was helpful*

here. The night nurses were also kind enough to allow me to stretch out on a gurney where I fell asleep instantly. It was possible to catch a couple of hours of sleep, but sometimes none.

However, this was one of my richest experiences. I was beginning to wonder if I really wanted to be a doctor. There were none in our family and I had so little idea of a doctor's life style that I could not realize what kind of preparation he needed.

Can we picture this life? The young man who viewed himself as a clumsy farm boy was struggling hard to master his subject, teaching Sunday School on his one day off and constantly attempting to respond to his family's need for his labor. Despite the challenges, Milo remained reflective on what he was doing.

I admired the head nurse and all that she knew. She had twenty years experience and knew illnesses, medicines and doctors—especially interns. One evening a severely injured man was admitted on the gurney. She sized up the situation as he came down the hall and went into her supply room to prepare for the emergency. One hour later when the interns had finished his history and physical examination, she was ready and had anticipated his every need. I read the history and it was very confusing. The man had been injured in a bakery and had told his story in bakery language which was plain to me because I had worked in a bakery, but not to the intern whose father had supported him in college and he had never worked anywhere. I decided then that a doctor needed to understand how people lived and worked in as many fields and lifestyles as possible. I decided then that I would work at as many different kinds of work as possible. The idea well fitted my financial status. Perhaps the admiration and respect I learned to have for nurses was my greatest gain.

Eventually Milo's exhaustion caused him to give the personnel director an ultimatum, and she agreed to let him split the job. When spring arrived, Milo was faced with paying off the $300 debt for his tuition. He was offered a teaching and coaching job in Robinson, Kansas for the coming autumn with a monthly check of $200, which would allow him to pay off the loan and begin saving again for the final years of medical school. That summer he worked for the Charles City Western Railroad.

> *I was given a job as helper to the shop foreman. It was a huge shop with train-size machinery. The foreman was a machinist of the old order and could manage all of it. We would bring an electric freight engine in and completely overhaul it. Make or turn new bearings throughout. Turn the drive wheels on the huge lathe to true up flat spots on the shoe. Or place an entire new rim on an engine or freight car wheel, true it on the lathe, and then case harden it. I learned to drive the big cars about the shop and freight yards and on weekends substituted on the road as a conductor or motorman or on slow days as both. It was a great learning experience.*

Today, Robinson, Kansas has a population of about two hundred people. When Milo began teaching there, the high school had about one hundred students. His job was to coach football, basketball and track, and to teach manual training and science subjects, such as agriculture and physiology or health science. He was the principal of six teachers.

> *Life was relaxed, peaceful and serene compared to the hard and long work hours in medical school. Maybe I didn't want to be a doctor after all. Teaching was rewarding.*

At the end of his first year, his contract was renewed with a ten-dollar a month raise, so he stayed. In the summer of 1927, Milo was intrigued by advertisements for athletic coaching courses, especially a six-week course in Madison, Wisconsin. He took a job as the night chef in a small café.

> *I slept in the car, shaved in the rear-view mirror and drove to breakfast and to classes, even in the rain . . . At the end I drove home to Charles City and had a good visit with Mother but was restless and wanted to travel, particularly to the west coast. I knew I could not afford to drive the Ford and keep it in repair, so I fixed a knapsack with a hammock of canvas for a bed and started to hitchhike about three one afternoon.*

Shortly he joined with five farm boys from Iowa who were taking a truck out to Washington State. "Jobs were divided: two serviced the car, two put up the tent, and they wanted me to help cook the meals." The adventures they shared began with an unexpected encounter.

> *The next day we were in the Black Hills at Rapid City and President Calvin Coolidge was taking a vacation there. We parked in front of the city library and waited for the parade and to glimpse the President. A large man came out of the library and visited with us on the steps. He said his name was Herbert Hoover. We had heard of his work with the starving Europeans at the end of WWI. He sat on the steps with us and watched the President go by.*

The first major breakdown of the truck occurred in the flat desert near Worland, Wyoming. Fearing rattlesnakes, Milo and the youngest of the boys slept on the top of the truck and were wakened "by the sun and a herd of curious wild horses." Following the horses on foot, Milo and the boy found themselves left behind by the others when they were offered a tow into the town, thirty miles away. Eventually, thirsty and foot-sore, the two were given a ride and reunited at a garage where they all waited for the repair.

> *We arrived in beautiful Yellowstone Park*

> *where we spent three days seeing all parts of the park. We had never before this trip seen mountains or bears or a high desert with prairie dog towns and wild horses.*

Arriving at their destination, the farm boys all got work. Milo joined a harvesting and threshing crew.

> *I was given a job of gathering the sacks of wheat from the field and hauling them to the elevator in the town. I had a four-horse team on a low frame wagon and had good exercise tossing the sixty-pound sacks on the wagon. I made two trips each morning and two in the afternoon and cared for the horses morning and night for which I was paid $5 per day. It was heavy but enjoyable work. Harvesting with such a huge combine was even more remarkable. The experience was a rich one and I felt added a new dimension to my life.*

School was to start in two weeks, so Milo headed south, finding a ride with a walnut farmer all the way to San Francisco. The two corresponded for the rest of their lives. At one point they waited by a huge redwood being cut by the side of the road. They measured one hundred yards of cleared trunk and were able to footrace one hundred yards side by side down the trunk.

> *I was awed by all the huge redwoods. Imagine me who had never even seen a tree until I was seven years old.*

Milo was unsettled by the rough characters in Carson City and asked a policeman for help. The officer put him up in the town jail, comfortably, and Milo then caught a ride with two dubious characters who took him across Wyoming and Nebraska, where he was befriended by a hobo who taught him how to jump a freight car. He was soon home.

> *It was a great change of lifestyle to dress-up and assume the duties of coach and principal in Rob-*

inson, Kansas. Now the situation I had so successfully avoided for many years took place: I was falling in love with Eva Crawford, the little dark-eyed music teacher of Everest, Kansas and we became engaged. She was not the outdoor rugged type nor missionary wife type, so I had to rearrange some priorities.

During the summer of 1927, Milo took a job in the Hart Parr tractor factory. His job was on the gangways of the molding floor where the castings were made. Although most of the loads were carried by two men, sometimes a sky hook was used. Once Milo's hand was caught by the sky hook, and he was hoisted in the air until the crane operator could lower him safely.

One job was scary. The core oven was a room that would hold a steel rack of many sand cores; 'cookies' they were called. In the center of the oven floor was the charcoal fire pit, about three feet wide, with a two foot shelf on either side, in which was a steel v-shaped trough that the roller supporting the racks rolled on. They would get filled with sand and debris and have to be swept out. The ledge was narrow, the air so hot that sometimes the broom caught fire and our breathing had to be shallow. It would be so easy to get dizzy and fall in the white hot pit.

It was heavy and exacting work. We wore, besides the felt skullcap with our ears tucked in, no shirt (all chest hair had been singed off), our trousers were moleskin without cuffs, pockets sewed up, shoes without laces, or if with laces, covered with clay. The reason for the dress was protection from the spattered molten iron. Sometimes it would even slop from the cauldron above. If the iron were white and liquid like water it would bounce harmlessly off our sweaty bodies or moleskin trousers. However, if the iron became cooled to red and stringy like syrup, it was very dangerous and could cut like a knife.

That autumn he returned to medical school and found jobs as a waiter and a janitor to pay for room and board. This was the year when Francis Peabody published his essay "The Care of the Patient" in JAMA 1927;88:877-882, in which he wrote:

> *the essence of the practice of medicine is that it is an intensely personal matter...The treatment of a disease may be entirely impersonal; the care of a patient must be completely personal. The significance of the intimate personal relationship between physician and patient cannot be too strongly emphasized, for in an extraordinarily large number of cases both diagnosis and treatment are directly dependent on it.*

This would be the creed of Milo's practice and later his daughter Donna's practice. She deeply grieves the passing of this understanding of the profession. But at the beginning, Milo was immersed in learning.

> *We saw patients every day and had many clinics to attend. There was less book studying and more observation. Everything varied from interesting to fascinating.*

Milo assisted at his own tonsillectomy. By mistake, he gargled with the hot alcohol put out for his back rub. This, however, stopped his throat from hurting and enabled him to return the next day to clinics and classes. The year passed quickly, and Milo relaxed by drawing up the plans to rebuild a home for his parents.

> *I had taught manual training and done considerable carpenter and building work, so I determined to try to see that Dad and Mother had a livable home free of mortgage.*

The house was well-constructed in 1884 when it had been built, but now it had to be raised on jacks and posts so that a basement could be dug and a proper foundation built. A mason was hired to build a new central chimney. Milo added as much new insulation as possible to the home, along with a new bathroom and tiling.

> *Total cost of the lumber and materials I had used was just over $1000 which Dad was able to pay besides the $350 cost of the chimney and plastering.*

> *Eva and I were engaged now; she came to spend a week with us while the house was on stilts and I was deeply absorbed in the building. She was at home in Cameron, Missouri for the summer, but teaching music in Corning, Iowa during the school year. She learned early about being ignored.*

Throughout the hundreds of pages of manuscript, there are very few descriptions of the women in Milo's life. We know that his mother was religious, frugal and constantly longing for a life of less discomfort and hardship. We know that Eva was a music teacher and that marrying her was, in Milo's view, the smartest thing he ever did. But we know surprisingly little more.

The senior year in medicine passed rapidly, and Milo graduated in 1930, eleven years after he had first entered college.

> *Graduation was June 2, after that I had Iowa State Board exams to take on June 3 and 4. On June 5th, Eva and I drove to the Clinton County seat at Plattsburg to get our marriage license. ... For me a big thrill was made possible by my sister Rena and her husband, Elgin Robeson, who drove some three hundred miles from Charles City, Iowa and brought my Mother, Melvina, and Dad, Ellsworth, along with my youngest brother, Walter (19) who served as my best man. Mother and Rena had become very fond of Eva when she had visited the summer before in Charles City. Mother was so pleased and proud to be there for the wedding of the fifth of her ten children, and*

> *thrilled that he had finally become a doctor. Dad had trouble believing it too.*

Choosing an internship was a challenge because most positions paid nothing, but finally, the Methodist Hospital of Southern California offered $25 per month besides room and board. The young couple would head west.

For Milo's father, Ellsworth, who had been born in the homesteader's sod house in Iowa and struggled constantly on the farm to make a life for his children and wife, Milo's graduation and marriage must have felt both extraordinarily fulfilling and at the same time lonely. The farm was gone, and now his companion for many years in the work of the farm was going west to California. The homesteading values had certainly brought the children from childhood to responsible adulthood, but Ellsworth knew that the world of the homestead had vanished.

As the young couple left to begin their lives together, Ellsworth and Melvina could hardly imagine what might lie ahead for them: it was and would be so different from what they had known. Yet if they had thought about the character of their son, they could have been confident: Milo was courageous, compassionate and willing to turn his hand to anything to help solve a problem. He had worked at hard and dangerous tasks and so knew the struggles of ordinary people. He was a patient observer, and a careful craftsman, both of which he had learned apprenticed to his father. With Eva he was ready for a new life.

Milo himself, decades later, wrote:

> *Looking back at it, almost fifty-two years ago, I can realize how little I appreciated the potential in happiness that that little dark eyed girl could bring to me in all these years.*

Chapter III

She Adjusted Early to Being Neglected

In the newspaper commentary on Eva and Milo's wedding, the editor wrote:

> *The bride is one of Cameron's most popular young ladies and is held in high esteem by all who know her. She possesses a very pleasing personality which has won for her a large circle of friends.*
>
> *After the three course wedding breakfast, Dr. and Mrs. Brooks left by auto for Los Angeles, California where they will be at home after July 1st.*
>
> *The Progress joins their many friends in wishing for them a happy and prosperous wedded life.*
>
> [rootsweb.ancestry.com]

Arriving for the internship year at Methodist Hospital of Southern California, the couple found a furnished apartment for $35 per month, but Milo's salary was just $25. Eva did not have a California teaching credential, so sought a secretarial job. Married women were not being hired, but after the intervention of friends and the removal of her treasured wedding ring, Eva was hired as "Miss Brooks". Milo was spending at least thirty-six hours out of every forty-eight at the hospital, one of four interns and one resident. Milo found a close, friendly group of colleagues and was quickly thriving, but for Eva it was a lonely time, with very rare outings to explore their new home.

> *The year was full of learning. Not only did we have excellent doctors practicing top quality medicine and surgery, but some not so good. And as Johnson, the cynical philosopher would say, it was a swell place to learn what not to do...*

> *Eva Danley, the excellent nurse from Seattle, made some Christmas cookies for Eva and me and as I stopped by to pick them up she looked awfully tired and was coughing badly. She said she had so much to do and they were having company for Christmas. The next day she entered the hospital on the medical floor where she had worked, with a diagnosis of pneumonia. Her breathing became difficult that night and the next morning as I came by her room she looked frightened and called for the supervising nurse who was very fond of her. Then she reached out her hand to me and said "Good bye". In another minute she was gone.*

What was the state of medicine in the 1930s that Milo called 'top quality'? The most common anesthetics were ether, chloroform and nitrous oxide, administered by the 'one drop' method on a cone held over the patient's nose. X-rays had been commonly used during World War I, and with the development of contrast medium, were used especially prior to surgery in most hospitals. The dangers of overexposure, or the therapeutic uses, were still unknown. Insulin was beginning to be used in general practice, but Milo complained of how little he knew of diabetes. There was no antibiotic available, and infectious diseases were treated primarily by isolation. Both tuberculosis and trichinosis (caused by worm-infested pork) were epidemic throughout the population. Courageous researchers, and crack-pots, were struggling to address the problems of cancer, of infection post-surgery, and of heart disease. Milo made a decision to stay near the rapid advances being made.

> *Too early in the intern year we had to decide if we wanted a residency. I had an idea that I would like to practice family medicine in some middle size city and felt the need of training in Pediatrics and Obstetrics, so applied for residency in each. I was accepted at Children's Hospital of Los Angeles. Also I was offered an OB residency; but since the Pedi-*

atric residency was difficult to get, I accepted it and thought I would take the OB the next year. But alas, when the time came, the OB people said they did not want a Pediatrician delivering babies. That ended my OB training.

During these years, Milo identified several teachers who would remain important mentors and friends throughout his life. Even as a senior professor, Milo would attend the staff conferences and evening X-ray reviews, striving to learn.

Conditions at the California Babies Hospital at the Lutheran Hospital were quite different but pleasant. The Pediatric ward had about twenty beds and there was also a sizable newborn service. There was also a large outpatient clinic called the Anita Baldwin Clinic. I was given complete charge of all three services, with excellent consultation from Drs. A.J. Scott and Earl Moody. However, they did not always make daily rounds and accepted my judgment unless I asked for help. I wouldn't have trusted me that much. The responsibility challenged me and I worked hard.

The Depression was affecting everything, but Milo's salary had increased to $50 a month, so the couple felt lucky.

I remember on Delongpre Avenue hearing a truck driver with a load of Valencia oranges calling, "Oranges, oranges, eighteen dozen for a quarter." I couldn't believe it and having a quarter, ran out on the street. Sure enough, he filled one laundry tray full and running over. We enjoyed lots of fresh oranges and orange juice. I could not help thinking of the poor orange farmer. It was too much like corn or potato failure.

In July of 1933, Milo and Eva moved to Westwood to a three-bedroom house. Milo made a sign "Milo B. Brooks,

M.D., Infants and Children" but no one came, so he continued to see patients for Dr. Scott. Eva was pregnant and had to give up work.

> *Dr. Earl Moody had just taken the position of Professor and Department Head at the College of Medical Evangelists at the White Memorial Hospital and offered me a job teaching in the clinic for $25 a month. I liked to teach and it would keep me up to date so I took it, but driving the fifteen miles each way every day used up most of the pay and most of my time. The only comfort we had was that no one else seemed to have any money either. It just seemed our lot was worse than most others. The long cherished dream of being a doctor and practicing in California was turning pretty bleak. Oh, I was alright, I was busy doing work I liked and getting free breakfast and lunch at the County hospital. But Eva had all day to think about the coming baby and what we would eat and how to pay our bills.*

On November 7, 1933, Donna Brooks was born, and Milo wrote: "Our little Donna was a beautiful plump healthy little girl and we could be quite happy." Donna's is the only birth mentioned in the memoir, the births of Richard and Ron are not referred to, and we have no other reference to Eva's worries about finances. Milo had now succeeded Dr. Moody as head of the Department of Pediatrics, his pay had been raised to $50 per month, and the college paid Milo's travels to other Departments of Pediatrics across the country.

> *I liked the students and in an attempt to get better acquainted, invited a section of fifteen to twenty at a time to spend an evening in our home in Westwood. This seemed to please and impress them and I enjoyed it too.*

Milo frequently brought unannounced guests home for a meal or an evening, no matter what was going on with Eva, who had simply to stretch the meals and accommodate these visitors. Donna comments "Mother was not a complainer," so we do not know how Eva felt about this, or the schedule that Milo kept.

> *My schedule was very demanding. I left home between 6 and 6:30 each morning, Monday through Friday and drove to the Los Angeles County General Hospital or White Memorial Hospital where I had breakfast and lectured and made rounds on patients until noon. Then I would drive to Westwood and see patients in the office until six or seven. Then I came home to eat the dinner which had been kept warm. There was no time to visit with Eva or the children as the phone was constantly ringing and I would answer three to six calls while trying to eat. Then there were house calls to make until ten or eleven o'clock, and after that lectures to prepare for the next day. This schedule lasted for twenty years, 1933-1953. ... My name was on every chart of about four to five thousand sick children each year and nearly an equal number of newborn and premature born.*

Donna learned to answer the telephone "Dr. Brooks' residence", but did not know what a residence was and had to explain to callers that she was too young to write a message. The one time when Eva and the children had Milo's undivided attention was early on Sunday morning. The family would drive to the beach at Santa Monica, and Milo would dig a large hole (complete with a bench) in the sand, and the children, giggling and laughing, would be temporarily buried up to their necks. This was the only place where the telephone did not interrupt the family. Then it would be home in order to go off to church, and Milo would again be rushing from one hospital to another. Just as it was during his years in medical school, building was a source of relaxation for Milo. On buying their first home, he immediately began carpentry projects.

> *First we cut a door in the back bedroom and built cement steps to enter the back yard. Next I built a picket fence and arched gate. Then built a [wooden] Jeep to scale, one quarter size. The boys had fun pushing it around the yard and sidewalks. Later I built a slide in the shape of an elephant and a sand box in the shape of a sail boat. Later I found a sturdy wooden crate about five feet square that was a shipping crate for an airplane motor. It made a nice playhouse especially after supporting each corner with a four by four post and elevating it eight feet off the ground and into our small willow tree. It had a narrow porch, a door, two windows, and a chimney of wood painted like bricks. A ladder on one support post furnished access, but I liked to grab the edge of the porch and swing my legs up onto the porch.*
>
> *Our back yard became the focal point for all the children in the block. Our children had much fun and many friends and the neighbors got relief from their children but it did add responsibility and care for Eva. Fortunately Mrs. Esther Bonner had a private school where our children were going and could use the elephant slide and sail boat sand box so there they served for several years.*
>
> *How did we manage tuition at private school? Mrs. Bonner was very kind to us and took the children in exchange for medical care at the school. I would take our three a little early and then examine each arrival as they came to try to isolate any early colds and try to prevent their spread in the school. Mrs. Bonner seemed to think it was worthwhile.*

Summer holidays for the family were paid for in the same way: Milo would take a *locum tenens* position as camp doctor, and Eva and the children would come with him and enjoy a change of scenery and camp activities. Often these were Boy Scout camps, as Milo also did the physical examinations for the Scouts who wanted to go to camp. The office at home in Westwood was not financially successful, so each additional way to support the family was eagerly accepted.

As soon as Donna was able to help, she was given jobs in the office. Milo as a father was just as he had been as a farm boy—an advocate of shared responsibility. Donna had to sterilize the glass syringes, fitting the plunger to the correct barrel after everything was clean. She also learned to sharpen the needles on a whet stone. When she was old enough she was allowed to help with patients, even once holding an infant while Milo drew off the fluid from the hydrocephalic child's brain. Sometimes, but not often, she would go to the hospital on rounds, though in an era of rampant polio epidemics, caution prevailed.

Then tragedy struck.

> *Right after Thanksgiving in 1940 when Donna was eight years of age, Richard five and a half and Ronald 3 we were living on Malcolm Avenue and my office was on Gayley Avenue where I had moved in 1937. Richard started with a headache and some vomiting. I was most concerned, and although I had not made a practice of treating our own children I decided to take Richard to the office and do a careful review of his history and a complete physical pretending to myself that he was a routine patient. My diagnosis was an intracranial expanding lesion. I jotted it down. It was very threatening as I remembered saying to myself when I had treated several brain tumors at Children's Hospital that that was the worst thing that could happen to any child.*

Richard spent a week at White Memorial Hospital, and the doctors assured Milo and Eva that he would get well. He came home for a few days, but his pain and vomiting recurred. He asked "Daddy, couldn't you please take me to a hospital where they don't have needles?" Milo's sister Delia and family arrived for a visit and were of great support. Suddenly early in the morning, the hospital called to say that Richard had taken a turn for the worse.

> *I found him in a coma and getting artificial respiration with a Bennett Machine.*

Soon he was transferred to the L.A. County Hospital, where a tank respirator [an iron lung] was available. The new neurosurgeon recommended immediate surgery and Milo consented.

> *Now his pulse became weak and suddenly stopped. I reached in and massaged his chest to no avail and after about ten minutes I called the operating room to cancel the surgery. It was a let down of tension, and I felt numb. I called Eva, who had been waiting all this time in the car, and we signed the permit for autopsy and headed for home.*
>
> *The office was scheduled full of patients and I needed something to do. The busy afternoon passed and I proceeded like a robot, feeling very sorry for myself, a doctor who couldn't save his own child. I wasn't very helpful to Eva or the children, but walked in a numb daze.*

The autopsy showed a cystic glioma in the left frontal lobe.

> *It seemed like I grieved a long time. In so doing I am sure I neglected Eva and the children who also had their grieving to do. I felt especially close to Ron, but somehow in feeling so sorry for myself, never did convey that feeling to him. My grieving instead made him feel that I cared more for Richard and was disappointed in him.*
>
> *I felt that if there was any good to come of this tragedy it was up to me to make it happen. I*

> *had thought that I was a caring physician, but now I would be more caring and go the second mile. So now when I stayed all night in the hospital for a very sick child, or when I took the suspected polio patient and his distraught parents to the hospital, instead of sending them, I could say to myself "This is for Richard."*

Milo's memoirs were written more than forty years after these events, but the pain, grief and guilt are palpable on the page. There is no comment on Eva's grief, or on how Donna and Ron dealt with the loss. Donna believes that both her mother and Ron blamed themselves for causing the tumor. Family pictures in Donna's album show a profound seriousness on her face in 1942, until the summer camp pictures with her cousins and friends. She is a serious pianist in one, looking guardedly at Ron—in another, her face, framed by dark curls, is not that of a child but of a very worried and aware person. When she was in fifth grade, Donna was ill with pneumonia which was treated with sulfa. She remembers the pills as "HUGE!"

Donna was now in public school and busy with Campfire Girls and church activities. Throughout WWII Milo substituted for other doctors and increased his time away from the family. Donna thought it terrible when he forgot to come home for dinner. Strikingly, Donna is often pictured holding a young animal—a goat, a puppy and feeding a deer in the Sequoias. The gentle touch that would make her beloved as a physician is obvious in the pictures. At one of the camps in the San Bernardino Mountains with her Campfire Girl friends, Donna was asked to direct the music, and when there was a fire, to keep the girls singing so that they would not be afraid. That, she recalls, was more successful than when she taught her campers to fish for trout. "They made sticks into fishing poles, I got line, and then we all tied on safety pins and threw them in the water." The experiment did not work.

With his constant travels across the country to medical meetings, Milo was able to stay in close touch with his siblings and their families. All of them grieved again together, as they had for Richard's death, when Maurice's son was killed in WWII. Although the larger family tried to gather together frequently, Westwood was filled with families with children, and Donna and Ron grew up with a close group of friends. Donna was looking toward college; Ron was taller than his sister.

The end of the war brought major changes to medicine. Milo was now at the top of his profession and ready to innovate.

Chapter IV

A Little Piece of God

Early in his residency in pediatrics, Milo had been profoundly affected by two patients.

> *One, a four year old boy, born without arms or legs, raced the other children by rolling. The other, was a nine year old girl with shortening of the upper portion of her right thigh. We call it proximal femoral focal deficiency PFFD now. She had about four inches of shortening and was able to ambulate rapidly by going up and down. No prosthesis was available at that time, and Dr. Steindler could find no surgery to improve her.*

In these early years, infectious diseases were rampant.

> *We had two afternoons a week when no other patients were seen but whooping cough. Those were noisy, busy afternoons. We had separate Ear, nose and throat, orthopedic, newborn and premature, well baby and pediatric surgical with attending men in those specialties. We even had a special mastoid clinic.*

Tuberculosis was a continual challenge. Mortality from these diseases was still over 20% per year for children under the age of five. Smallpox vaccination was required to protect the public's health. The Diphtheria, Pertussis and Tetanus vaccines were combined in 1948 as DPT and used widely. Measles and rubella were still causing widespread epidemics. In 1964-65, over twenty thousand cases of rubella occurred, leaving large numbers of children blind, deaf or with mental retardation. Trying to establish a pediatric practice, Milo had to be extra cautious about all these risks. Sometimes on a house call, he would paint a child's throat, one of the few hands-on interventions known to be effective against diphtheria. He carried with him in his medical bag a small hand puppet monkey, named Bosco, which would come out to engage and distract the child and evoke at least a tentative smile.

But other challenges of clinical work were equally daunting.

> *In my private practice started in the depth of the depression of the 1930's I had a great empathy for people without money. I decided to see if it was possible to see that no patient who sought my medical care should not receive it because of inability to pay. Anyway I had not studied medicine with the idea of making money.*
>
> *In addition I was flattered to have the students and faculty first from USC, then Loma Linda, and later UCLA bring their children to me without charge. Through the twenty-five years of my private practice that averaged one third of my practice.*

A pattern had been established:

> *Starting the Child Amputee Prosthetics Project at UCLA (1952) we decided to apply the same principle of not refusing care for reason of inability to pay to that program. Fortunately, the California Crippled Children's Service was very interested in this project and able to fund nearly all of the needs. The few children not covered by CCS Insurance or parents capable of paying were taken care of by funds obtained from the Junior Chamber of Commerce, Women's Clubs or service clubs. Now after twenty-nine years of the Child Amputee Project we are able to say that over twelve hundred limb deficient children have been fitted with all the equipment the project felt they needed regardless of ability to pay.*

That is my legacy in lieu of a life savings.

Today we might wonder how this was possible, for we live in a time when very few doctors make such decisions. It is clear that Milo felt such choices were his responsibility, and an aspect of the care he was giving. From his earliest years in practice, Milo wanted to find ways to improve the outcomes for the patients and their families. At the Los Angeles County Hospital, the premature infant project, which Milo directed even during his residency saw the death rate cut in half. He argued for everything from screens on the windows to keep out insects to different ways of handling the tiny newborns. Then there was polio.

> *The big polio epidemic of the late thirties brought a lot of patients to the Contagious Disease Center at the Los Angeles County Hospital. All of our residents rotated through this service and it was a favorite. I became somewhat acquainted with the service through the residents although my attending service had been earlier, when there were wards full of diphtheria cases. My criticism was largely the lack of personal concern for the anxious patients and their parents.*
>
> *Few people now can imagine the terrors of those years, when children could be laughing and playing in the afternoon, and struggling for breath, paralyzed perhaps for life, the next day.*
>
> *Running well baby clinics before starting office practice gave me some lasting experiences. In one clinic two mothers refused to allow immunization even after I had carefully explained the advantages and risks. One was afraid of 'foreign' materials and the other did not think it necessary. On my service at contagious diseases at LA County I was to see both of these children die of diphtheria. It was a horrible and wrenching experience.*

> *I did decide that I would not continue to care for a patient in my private practice whose parents refused immunization. I did lose a few patients at a time when I desperately needed every patient, but I never did give in. I never did need to review my patients to see who was immunized.*

Now, in 2013, immunization rates in the United States have stagnated at a mere 82% of children, in part because immunizations are not free in a public health program. The Centers for Disease Control also reports that immunization rates for adults for most of the common infectious diseases are very low, and that four out of five children who suffered from whooping cough (now again epidemic) caught it from an older member of the household. One out of every five children who contract measles will require hospitalization for complications, yet some parents still argue that the risks from the vaccination are more that the risks of contagion. Milo would have little patience for such a view.

> *"I had large mirrors back of each examining table to watch myself in handling a small child; also to watch the parents' reaction. It is so easy if you don't watch to handle a child like a sack of flour or even be rough with uncooperative children. One child had tried my patience and I decided to try extreme gentleness to avoid hurting him. He responded and cooperated beautifully. The father remarked "Doctor, you held our boy like he was a little piece of God."*

> *Years later at the Child Amputee Prosthetic Project when we discovered that the parents' attitude was the most important single factor in the proper adjustment of a limb deficient child, we decided to try to induce a positive attitude before others were formed. By visiting the child and parents in the hospital on the day of birth or soon after, the first examination in the presence of the parents was most*

effective. The infant could be held like he was a real person and most worthwhile, even if he looked like little broken pieces of God.

Milo the carpenter made his examination tables and other furniture, but that was not all.

On house calls, often for acute febrile conditions, a painful injection of penicillin was needed. I searched for a way to ease the painful memory if not the pain. I learned to make tiny animals like dogs and rabbits out of pipe cleaners. These were effective if made with the child watching, after the shot was given and apprehension relieved. It seemed to give them something to remember me by besides the shot.

Early in 1941, Milo was one of nine doctors who wanted to build an office and practice location together. Milo helped develop the plans, but after Pearl Harbor all building permits were suspended, so when the building was completed, it had to be a cheaper version.

We kept the building from 1945 to 1965, renting the six suites and paying the same rent ourselves. Our main advantage was having a building arranged according to our desires and no foreign landlords. Those were very busy years with teaching half days at LA County and White Memorial Hospitals and then putting in a full day in the office. I was tired of commuting.

The College of Medical Evangelists was changing, and Milo recommended that the position of head of the department should be full time not half time. Although they offered him the post, Milo was also offered a full professorship at UCLA and the chance to develop what became his child amputee project.

I decided to change schools rather than home and place of business. Thus ended twenty delightful

> *years of association with the [Loma Linda] College of Medical Evangelists. They made me an Honorary Life Member of the Hospital Staff.*
>
> *In 1958 The California Crippled Children's Services who were financially sponsoring the project requested a full time medical director, and asked me to give up my private practice to come as a full time director and full professor at UCLA.*
>
> *I was reluctant to give up my practice as now I had a very dependable assistant in Dr. Leslie Holve, and had worked out an exchange of calls with four other pediatricians in the area so that we could have some evenings free of calls. I was most fortunate to have someone as competent and agreeable as Les with whom to leave my practice. It was a great satisfaction to leave my patients in his good hands. Also it was good at sixty years of age to have eight hour days and five day weeks. It seemed more like retiring than when I really did retire at eighty-three in 1981.*

Milo at this time was a proficient professional, but he was restless about the profession itself.

> *The reason I wanted something in interdisciplinary work was because I felt that we as physicians had specialized so much that we had left the patients to fall between the cracks. I felt that my pediatric training would help me be the 'patient's advocate' and add that personal touch so needed when a patient and their family are surrounded by a group of specialized professionals. That role I tried to play in the twenty-eight years I was with the Child Amputee Prosthetic Project. It was a role I enjoyed.*

More than fifty years later, Milo would hardly recognize the specialization today as 'care', and would no doubt be shocked that specialists do not talk with each other, let alone with the non-physicians who interact with the patient.

> *All other amputee projects in the country were administered in an Orthopedic Department or at least in Rehabilitation medicine, but at UCLA it had been decided that all projects dealing with children should be administered in the Pediatric Department. The staff consisted of Orthopedists, Psychologists, Psychiatrists, Engineers, Medical Social Workers, Occupational and Physical Therapists and Prosthetists, or limb makers.*

> *Decisions made by the staff were to treat the whole child in addition to his limb deficiency and substitutes. His general health, diet, exercise, immunizations, school and the emotional needs of him or her and their parents. We went to the hospital soon after birth to help parents cope with the shock and tell them what they could expect and not expect.*

The brochure on the project is a model of good sense and great appeal. It begins:

> *What is a limb deficient child? A child who has one or more limbs missing is a child who likes to play, a child who attends a neighborhood school, a youth who looks forward to a career and family.*

All the years of building and the many skills used decades before on the farm came into play, as Milo worked with engineers and prosthetists to address the needs of his patients.

One of the most challenging aspects of medical practice remains that of giving answers to parents, especially when there may be no acceptable answers.

> *We sought to study the cause of limb birth defects as every parent asks 'why' and we can only answer 'God only knows'. We analyzed all the*

cases born in hospitals in Southern California over twenty years, but got little insight. Then when the Thalidomide episode occurred in Europe in 1961 with 4000 deformed children in Germany alone, I was anxious to see this thing.

Before the journey to Europe could take place, however, Eva and Milo had decided to move to a new home. Donna was practicing as a physical therapist and was enrolled to start medical studies at the Women's Medical College of Pennsylvania. Ron was living in San Francisco with a thriving furniture shop while he took courses in anthropology.

We had lived at Holman Avenue for seventeen years and had always liked the place where we had spent so many happy days. We found a house on a hill with a view overlooking Westwood and out on to the ocean. Moving day came and went smoothly. One thing about the new house bothered me. It had a shake shingle roof and was in a fire hazard area. I rigged up a rainbird sprinkler system to cover the whole house with a valve that turned on in a closet off the hall.

We had been living there six weeks when on November 6, after I had thought the fire hazard was over we had a dry period and a warm Santa Ana wind that blew all night. I went to the project at UCLA to work that morning, our insurance agent called to say our new policy was in force and did I know there was a small fire about two miles from us. I called Eva and she said everything was fine and she was doing some washing. A half hour later she called and said I'd better come. I left in a few minutes and it takes about ten minutes to drive, but I was about six blocks from home when I met Eva. She said "Turn around and come with me. Don't go in there, it's a holocaust." Those glad moments when we met on that road make it difficult for me to feel sad about anything else.

Friends took them in, and they spent an anxious night wondering what was happening.

> *We drove up to find our house completely gone to the foundations and chimney. The frame of our little grand piano was lying under what had been the living room. There was no sign of the porcelain bathroom fixtures and the porcelain lined steel bath tubs had melted. We felt worst about the piano, the solid walnut bed my grandfather had made, our antique spinning wheel and grandmother's Seth Thomas clock."*

In the 1961 Bel Air Brentwood fire, as it came to be called, 484 homes were lost, fifty of them in Milo and Eva's neighborhood. They moved into a small apartment until it was time to leave for the European trip. In the meantime, all the Brooks siblings were concerned about the fire. Milo wrote them a combined letter:

> *It is not because we are brave that we have not complained; we simply are so well taken care of and comfortable that there is little to say. How two people can lose so much and be so little inconvenienced for comfort and necessities is hard to realize. At first the shock was so rapid, complete and irrevocable that there was nothing to fight back at or worry over. As time goes on one looks for things or thinks of something that is gone and the impact gradually sinks in and deepens.*
>
> *There has been a neighborliness and comradeship among the refugee residents out of this disaster. The street will soon be rebuilt and be more beautiful than ever.*
>
> *Our Christmas was one of the nicest and happiest we have had Donna and Ronnie were both home. Vincent and Cindy (Ron's children) were there*

too and they are both old enough to get the most out of Christmas and presents.

Ronnie did a nice thing for us. We had not planned a Christmas tree for this small apartment but he thought we should. So one night after we had gone to bed he slipped across the street to a tree lot for a tree then got decorations of gold ornaments, lights, and strung cranberries and popcorn to surprise us the next morning.

A year ago when we were looking at houses Eva wanted to move into a nice new home all built, I wanted to find a lot to build on as we pleased. Now we both have our wish, but I guess I shouldn't have wished so hard. We have an ideal New Year's situation with all the things of the past burned away and a whole new future to look forward to.

This is clearly the same Milo who watched the prairie burn as a child and knew that life must move forward.

The European trip began with a standard two-week tour, and then Milo and Eva were able to spend another two weeks visiting with friends and colleagues and consulting with the orthopedists and prosthetists who worked with the thalidomide children. When they returned, the Westwood Village Rotary Club asked Milo to talk about the trip. The UCLA publicity manager asked if he would answer questions from the press.

When I arrived there were six television stations crowding their equipment in the parking lot and twelve newspaper reporters. A news conference was held in the adjacent room and it made national evening television news. My little mother in Iowa was ecstatic when she saw her son on the television news each hour. She really thought her little troublesome boy had finally arrived.

Over the next several years, Milo reviewed many x-rays and made many depositions over thalidomide and the impact on children. Here is one of his most telling comments made in regard to taking statements from the children themselves:

> *I wish to note that when a person accentuates and perpetuates their disability, whether to win sympathy or a court case, they inevitably lessen their chance for rehabilitation and a more normal life.*

Despite their fears of fire, Milo and Eva moved into another house with a shake shingle roof, but were able to live there happily for nineteen years. In 1965, UCLA was trying to enforce their compulsory retirement policy; Milo found Yoshio Setoguchi to take over the prosthetic project in 1967.

> *He hired me back as a consultant so that I would continue seeing patients but without administrative duties. This continued to 1981 when I finally retired at 83. Yosh has carried the Child Prosthetics Project to new heights of excellence.*

Writing about the amputee program after its first three years of operation, Milo outlined the critical points, which are as contemporary today for the care of children—and adults—as when it was written in 1956:

"1. Team effort for involved rehabilitation problems seems to be more effective than any other approach.

2. Psychological effect on both the patient and family is much deeper than was realized.

3. The optimum age for first fitting of a prosthesis is much earlier than had been generally believed—under one year, as opposed to age five or later.

4. Training adequate for efficient and easy use of the prosthesis is absolutely essential and must be followed with periodic training in new skills.

5. Comfort and function must be provided or a prosthesis will not be used.

6. Scaled-down adult components are helpful, but do not supply all the needs of growing children. Special types of tools are needed for the many varied activities of childhood.

7. At the outset of the program, disability was calculated in terms of the site of amputation. Now it is realized that the true determination of disability is above the ears."

When Milo studied medicine, and when he began his internship in 1930, fifty-one years before his retirement in 1981, there were few effective treatments for infectious diseases; a physician had few tools for technical diagnosis or intervention and therefore relied on observation and judgment. The trust between a physician and patient was viewed as inviolate and as having an essential and immeasurable impact on healing and health. He saw wards full of children with diphtheria and held a special whooping cough clinic, in addition to seeing the first iron lung developed for use—beyond hot packs—with polio patients. By the time he retired, he had not only witnessed the impact of the vaccines for these diseases, but had introduced first penicillin and then other antibiotics as they became available.

He had begun teaching even before he had an independent practice and continued to teach throughout his life. He was trying to train his students to pay attention to what he felt was a holy and sacred calling. Having been raised in the hard apprenticeship of farming and direct apprenticeship in medical school, he viewed all of his students as apprentices in a calling which was both a supremely skilled craft and a supremely spiritual dedication.

In 1990, at the Association of Children's Prosthetic and Orthotic Clinical Meeting, Ernst Marquardt, orthopedic surgeon of Heidelberg, told this story of Milo Brooks:

The doctor walked through the clinic,
And saw a mother apart from her child,
A limbless child, propped and estranged:
A woman afraid to touch,
Far from loving.
He detoured, directly to the baby
And picked it up, enfolding it,
Cradling it to his chest,
And loving, loving.
"What a beautiful baby you have!"
to the wide-eyed woman.
He patted again, admired,
And gave the child to the mother, barrier-breaking.
Back in the office he told the team
"You can't just wait to send for the psychologist."
The Pediatrician (Milo Brooks, By Ernst Marquardt)

Milo's mother was interviewed by a newspaper on the occasion of her sixty-eighth wedding anniversary. Her advice on how to stay married was "Learn patience and be understanding," which was essentially Milo's advice to his students.

As he and Eva travelled extensively during the years of retirement, they visited with these students, and with the many Rotary exchange students they had welcomed into their family. The time had come for reflection, which Milo approached with the same rigor and determination that he had shown since, with pride at age of ten, he said, “I was glad to be trusted with a man’s job.”

Chapter V

Just Keep Going

In May of 1972, the Westwood Village Rotary Club surprised Milo and Eva by a "This is Your Life" celebration. The stories told traced Milo's adventures from the struggles to get through medical school to his years teaching and the founding of the UCLA Medical School in 1946. Further, to his becoming head of the Department of Pediatrics at Loma Linda, and as a culmination, the establishment of the Child Amputee Prosthetic Project. What was unique about this day was the emphasis placed on Milo's involvement in the Boy Scouts of Westwood, the YMCA and its physical fitness program, the Rotary International Exchange Student Program, and Westwood Community Methodist Church.

Despite the schedule of his clinical care, Milo's life was embedded in his community and in his service to that community.

> *Lew Stroh, one of our newer members and now Director of the Westside Family YMCA spoke briefly about Milo in the ten years he has known him. For many years Milo has worn a tiny rose bud in his lapel. On the morning that Lew was to be interviewed by the Board of Directors for the job Milo showed up a little early and pinned a rosebud on Lou's lapel saying 'Maybe this will bring you good luck.' Lew said, "And it did—I got the job and he brought me a rosebud for every board meeting he attended after that.*

Fifteen years later, May 7, 1987, was also Milo Brooks Day at Westwood Village Rotary Club, and a plaque was presented in honor of the "forty-four years of Service Above Self" the motto of Rotary.

Maurice, Milo's older brother, had started writing down his memories to share with his siblings, and at the end of 1965 Milo commented to him that these stories told him things he had never known, for instance that Maurice and his mother learned to read and write English together while speaking French.

Perhaps it was Maurice's efforts which encouraged Milo to begin writing, or the *Brooks Babbler*, the round-robin newsletter which the siblings began circulating in 1934 which reinforced both ties and a sense of obligation to the shared tradition. It stopped circulation in 2012, after over 78 years of family contribution. The comments in the *Babbler* are not only on the events of various family members and their lives, but on the communities in which they lived and worked. Milo often comments on medical issues, and particularly as his siblings age, he explains their ailments and treatments to them in the newsletter. Rena especially keeps everyone informed of who is doing what where, and takes delight in keeping her brothers from forgetting their roots.

Many of the travels undertaken in these years were prompted by a medical conference, but concluded with Milo and Eva seeking out family members and conducting extensive genealogical research. In 1979, for instance, they attended a conference on the "Mechanisms of Growth Control" where Milo was fascinated by the use of electric and magnetic stimulation on cell growth. At the end of the academic meeting, they drove from Syracuse to Oswego, New York, where Milo's mother had been born. They found the office of history in the Chenango County Museum and went through various census books, finding that a Daniel Brooks, born in 1765 left Connecticut to buy land in 1807.

Eva enjoyed searching through the old cemeteries. Several of the Brooks siblings must have devoted hundreds of hours to genealogical research, for the family papers trace back to 1591 to the birth of one Henry Brooks who then settled in Massachusetts around 1630. Milo's sisters, Rena and Julia did the bulk of the early work.

Milo wrote to Donna, busy in her OB/Gyn practice, in sending her these early records:

> *You may notice that Henry's second wife Suzanna was apparently a midwife known as Goodwife Brooks. However, she is not a blood ancestor.*

As the memoirs took shape, and as Milo saw his students become successful professors around the world, he reflected more on his own temperament.

> *Dr. Rogne preached a sermon on what to do when you are discouraged or despondent. I can't ever remember being either discouraged or despondent. Maybe I took such things as crop failure, lack of money, Richard's death and the fire too lightly. But I think I was just looking beyond. What do you think?*

Men and women of Milo's generation, especially those who came from farming roots, made their lives, and our nation, by 'just looking beyond'. Life was filled with challenge and sorrow, but there was little point in complaint. In the face of prairie fires, infant deaths, the Great Depression and financial struggles, they viewed their most important task to be the next step forward.

From the perspective of 2013, they may seem unemotional– and certainly, they were rarely given to verbal outbursts about their feelings or their moods. Most of them, like Milo, were simply too busy, too driven and absolutely committed to doing something positive rather than feeling or saying something positive. It was action they valued.

Yet we know from Milo's Memoirs that he was profoundly distraught over Richard's death, and his own inability to help his son, and then, his family. Donna does not view her father's busy life as neglect, she says he was simply otherwise occupied and could not make time for either the children or for his wife. As we read the writings of the siblings in the *Brooks Babbler*, hardship is not viewed as suffering. They offer each other sympathy and concern over human tragedies, but they do not rage or blame anyone for the tragedies.

On the occasion of his eighty-sixth birthday, Milo and his family went to church. At the luncheon afterward, where he was presented with a large card, the minister asked him "Would you like to say something and tell us how you attain this age?"

> *He handed me the microphone and I said "You just keep on going."*

At home that evening, Milo thought of what he might have said and wrote it down:

> *Dr. Rogne you explained to us this morning in your sermon how we are not promised a rose garden. But I have a rose garden, though not ever deserving it. These eighty-six years have been wonderful and I have enjoyed every one that I can remember.*
>
> *The loveliest bloom in my rose garden is Eva. You all know Eva, can you imagine the pure joy of living fifty-four years with a loving and caring person like Eva. Our cup runneth over.*
>
> *And that is not all, we have two wonderful children. My grandfather Daniel Brooks was a skilled craftsman, a wagon-maker by trade but he built barns and houses and could fix anything that broke on the farm, and it often did. My father was like that too, he built houses and barns and repaired*

more complicated farm machinery.

I tried to be a fixer like that too, but our Ron is the true craftsman. Everything Ron puts his hands on comes out beautiful. . . . That is not all, Ron has two children that are very special to their grandparents.

Some of you know our Doctor daughter Donna. People often say "Aren't you proud that your daughter is a Doctor?" Well, No! But I am bursting my buttons because of the kind of caring Doctor she is. She is a knowledgeable and skillful surgeon too. She has earned the respect of her colleagues and is President of the San Diego Gynecology Society.

So you see, our cup runneth over and over and we do have a rose garden.

Such personal expressions of love and pride are very rare, not only in Milo's writings, but for his generation. Known as an exceptionally loving physician, Milo had many ways to express his warmth with every patient, but for the family the other statement was apt: "You just keep on going."

In another note, a year later Milo wrote to Donna:

It was so good of you to drive all the way up here and back just to make my Day. I was proud to have you meet so many of our friends. We love you.

And Eva: "Thank you so much for coming, it made our day complete, but so sorry you were so tired. Love, Mother and Pappy"

As often as they could, the Brooks siblings gathered together. For some years these reunions had been to celebrate their parents' long marriage, but the family carried on meeting together for over three decades after their parents died. Melvina died in 1956, Ellsworth in 1958. They had been married for seventy-one years. Despite having less than five years of schooling between them, they raised their nine children to be educated and contributing citizens. Never prosperous in a material sense, they exemplified a commitment to community, and a Biblical morality of duty, rectitude and service to others typical of homesteading families, but rare in our contemporary society.

In June of 1983, seventy-six members of the extended Brooks family assembled in Dubuque, Iowa, one hundred and sixteen years after Daniel Brooks had homesteaded nearby. After the two-day gathering Milo and Eva and Donna were taken on tours of various family farms. Milo the pediatrician was now seeing how farming had changed since he walked behind his team of horses:

> *I was interested to see that the beef stock was selected by computer records on such traits as size at birth, at 160 days and mothering efficiency of the cow. Mixed breeds were preferred over thoroughbreds.*
>
> *The pastures were farmed by being leveled and cleared of rocks. John's farm is on the terminal glacial moraine. Then the area is cultivated and a specially planned grass seed mixture sown that produces two to three times as much forage as native grasses.*

They visited the homestead and the home where eight of the ten Brooks children were born. Milo had thought the round barn would stand for ever, but after seventy years the shingles were gone from the roof and some of the brick tile had cracked. Milo wanted to set to work to repair it. They then went from Nassau to Charles City twelve miles away "It was such a long way when we drove it with horses." During the trip they were able to visit the model farms from 1850 forward, and Milo felt right at home. Moving south to Kansas City, Missouri, they now attended the Crawford family reunion where over fifty family members gathered.

Afterward, Milo wrote:

> *Donna you did a super job of typing up and correcting the reunion's notes and fast too. I have gone over them and find little to change except that I seemed to neglect personal reference to some of the deserving 'Crawfords'.*
>
> *I love you, your Dad.*

The warmth of this note is reassuring, for Donna had faced a very hard decision in that year. Milo was still examining children and consulting at the Prosthetics project at UCLA, despite his increasing deafness. Finally, in the interest of patient safety, Donna took away his stethoscope, and told her father that he must no longer use it because he could not hear with any accuracy. This took great courage and in fact precipitated Milo's final 'retirement' from patient care. That she took this step speaks both to Donna's integrity as a physician, and to her dutiful and loving regard for her father.

Increasingly now, Milo, at eighty-five, and Eva were dependent on Donna's concern and attention. It was soon necessary for her to take away his drivers' license as well, and he resented becoming dependent but respected her judgment.

The surviving Brooks siblings were still keeping alert to each other, even though by 1980 the nine had become three and it was the second generation that continued gathering. Some of the family struggled at times to keep up with the changing world. Maurice, retired in Florida, did not miss the hardships of the early days. Ruby, who taught classes in reminiscence writing, comments wryly:

> *Good luck with your computer. They have their own personalities, I think, some good, some mischievous, some downright mean.*

Everywhere Milo and Eva travelled, Milo met with pediatricians. In February of 1981 Donna took them to Maui to celebrate their fiftieth wedding anniversary the year before, and immediately upon their return they were visited by Ernst Marquardt from Germany.

> *I enjoyed the days with him. He came to our Project each day and discussed cases. He is the most famous orthopedist in Europe and has the largest Children's Amputee clinic in the world.*

When they attended the meeting of the Southwest Pediatrics Society, Milo conducted the clinic for amputee children at the San Diego Children's Hospital. Eva had enjoyed the genealogy trips and reunions, and was discovering that she also enjoyed the international journeys, eventually seeing the South Seas, New Zealand, the Middle East, and most of Europe. Milo and Eva even took an immersion Spanish course in Mexico when both were in their eighties.

When they were first engaged, Milo thought that Eva would not want the life of a missionary and attributed his abandonment of that goal to his choice of bride. In later life, Eva truly enjoyed travels, and there are many pictures of her looking happy and relaxed in some foreign city. Because she is largely invisible in Milo's penned memoirs, it is easy to forget that Eva was a college-educated woman in an era when few women were, and that Milo's ability to lead the life he chose depended upon her ability to sustain the home and family without much attention from him.

Milo was often asked to give a eulogy, or speak at the funeral of a contemporary. The farm boy from the sod house sometimes sounded awestruck by the famous people he met. In one eulogy he mentioned being introduced to the author of *The Nun's Story*, and then said "We also met the Nun." Another Brooks reunion took place in 1985 in California, with Milo doing much of the organization beforehand.

Although Milo was not greatly interested in the administration of medicine, his curiosity, time-management and organizational skills made him a natural researcher. In his early years he had wanted to find a better way to care for premature infants and built cages for opossums in the backyard in order to study the marsupial care. Eva disdained the smell and the mess.

In the prosthetics project, Milo undertook a study of salamanders in order to watch the limb growth and monitor the effects of various interventions. In these final years, especially in his correspondence with family members, Milo seems at times to view aging as yet another research project. In 1982 the book on the Limb Deficient Child had been republished, and as he corresponded about the memoirs and the family, Milo frequently asked how the Brooks family history might be organized in a logical way.

Ron, who was living at home with his parents, and Milo were doing the cooking and much of the housekeeping. Ron had struggled at times with drug addiction and clinical depression as well as debilitating pain. Donna does not recall being aware of a precipitating event, but she feels that Eva's functioning was deteriorating in the early stages of the Alzheimer's disease which would dominate the rest of her life. Ron had throughout his life been dependent on his parents at various times, and he was now fully moved in to the guest bedroom.

At the end of January, 1986, all things changed again. Ron had suffered from ankylosing spondylitis, a disease of the spine which causes chronic pain. He was trying to learn to manage the pain but was unable to accomplish his beloved woodworking. On the 31st of January, Ron shot himself. Milo found him and called Donna who immediately headed north to her parents. Ten months later, Milo wrote to the family:

> *You all know of Ron's death on January 31*
> *and of our own grief and struggle with this tragedy.*

> *We have been of little help to Donna, Vincent and Christine, Cindy and Lisa. Just now we are completing transforming his room into a guest bedroom. He had collected so many things. I took back about one hundred pounds of library books he had recently borrowed from the UCLA library. There were fifteen boxes of Anthropology books that went to his memorial library at the Southwest Museum and there are five more to go. It seemed we had to stop and cry a little so very often.*

In an effort to recover from the grief and from a lingering flu-like illness which was severe, Eva and Milo took a cruise to Alaska in the summer of 1986. Donna now believes that neither of her parents ever really recovered from Ron's death. For Milo, the guilt he felt over not having been able to help Richard was compounded by his guilt over Ron's suicide. There were very few distractions from that internal sorrow, but they were both thrilled by the Alaskan scenery, but found their stamina greatly reduced. Visitors and the extended family kept coming, but in January of 1987, Donna was alarmed by her father's shortness of breath. He spent over three weeks in hospital in San Diego, while Eva moved into a retirement community near Donna's home. By March, with Milo in a wheelchair, the furniture was moved from Westwood into their retirement cottage. Eva's sight was failing, so both were grateful for the new comfort and convenience. Milo gave the facility his highest praise "The library is excellent and the woodworking shop has more equipment than I had at home." He did of course start attempting to repair the entire building to his standards.

Donna wrote to the *Brooks Babbler*:

> *The folks are doing well in their new location, though the transition was forced by illness. The freedom of maintenance and meal preparation responsibility makes a lot of difference. Entertaining guests is quite easy and lots of their friends have come by.*

> *Daddy has been learning the bus routes and getting out quite a bit. Mother keeps their cottage neat and homey as ever.*

On the night of June 7, 1987, Milo went to bed as usual and died in his sleep. Eva, sadly diminished by Alzheimer's and glaucoma, was lovingly cared for by Donna until her death on February 19, 1992.

Milo Brooks lived the arc of the American dream: from the struggles in a sod house on the prairie to three professorships and leadership of his profession to comfort and contentment and time to reflect. It is significant that Milo was never interested in the financial rewards of medicine, and both practiced and lived his life in terms of service. We can marvel that he found time to be a contributing member of his church, to Rotary and the YMCA, as well as to all the aspects of teaching and innovation in pediatrics. If we judge the contribution to the profession and community in terms of the cost to Eva and to the family, we would also judge his generation. Those who worked through the Depression and then those who served in WWII shared a commitment to purpose, to meaningful action. Their values emphasized the public context of their lives, not their private concerns.

We have to remember that farm children from their earliest years were in an apprenticeship through which they learned both skills and attitudes. We see that Milo carried on that tradition in his willing engagement of Donna as a young child in the daily duties of his practice. He apparently also tried to engage Ron similarly, but for reasons unknown to Donna, the two never were able to work companionably. However, Milo did have students from his earliest years in medicine and tried always to teach the sense of calling and respect for the person who was temporarily a patient. He consciously saw himself as a steward of a tradition.

If we think of the journey from homestead to hospital professorships, we must also remember that Milo and Eva wanted "something positive to do, not just something positive to say." The enormous record of their lives in the *Brooks Babbler* and in Milo's memoirs is part of the legacy of invisible strength that might be forgotten, or taken for granted, were it not for the next part of the story.

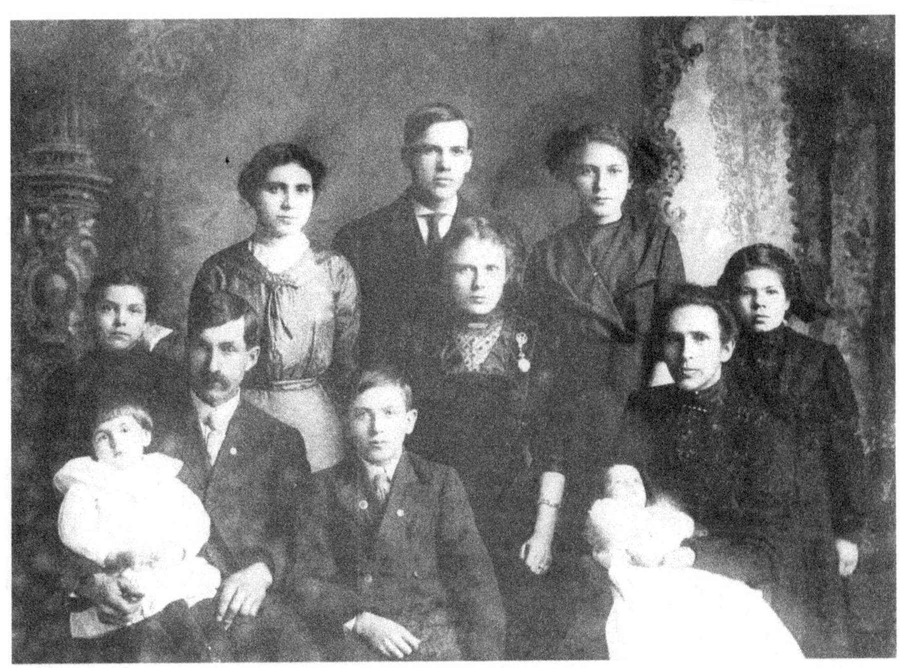

EE. Brooks Family in 1911

Left to Right Standing

Julia, (10), Delia (22), Maurice (24), Rena (19), Frances (16),

Evelyn (11)

Seated

Leroy (2), Father EE. Brooks (48), Milo (13), Mother Melvina (43), holding Walter (3 months)

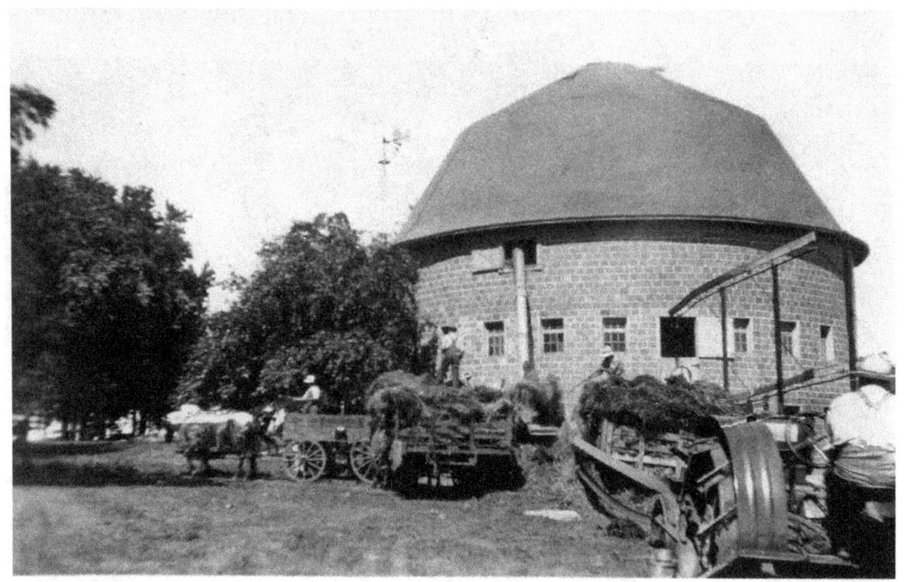

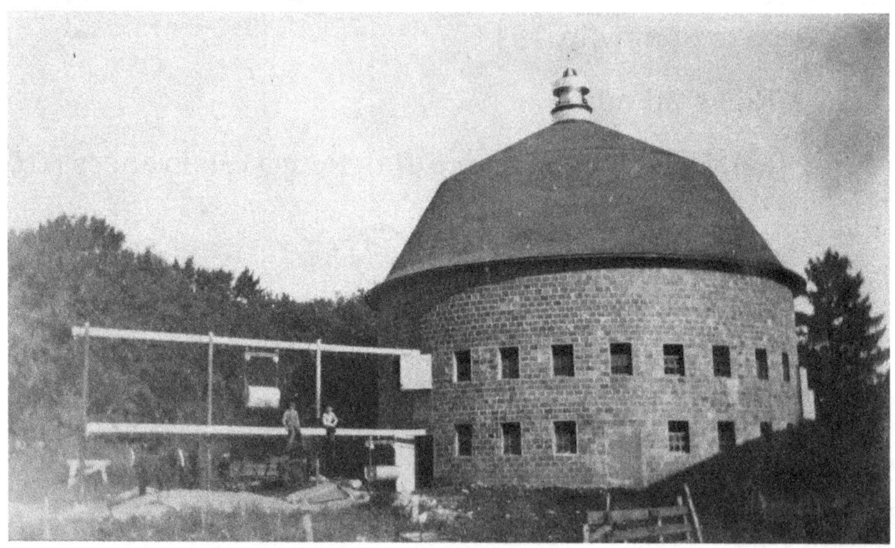

The Round Barn 1914

Upper picture: under construction '
Lower Picture: completed, it stood for 81 years

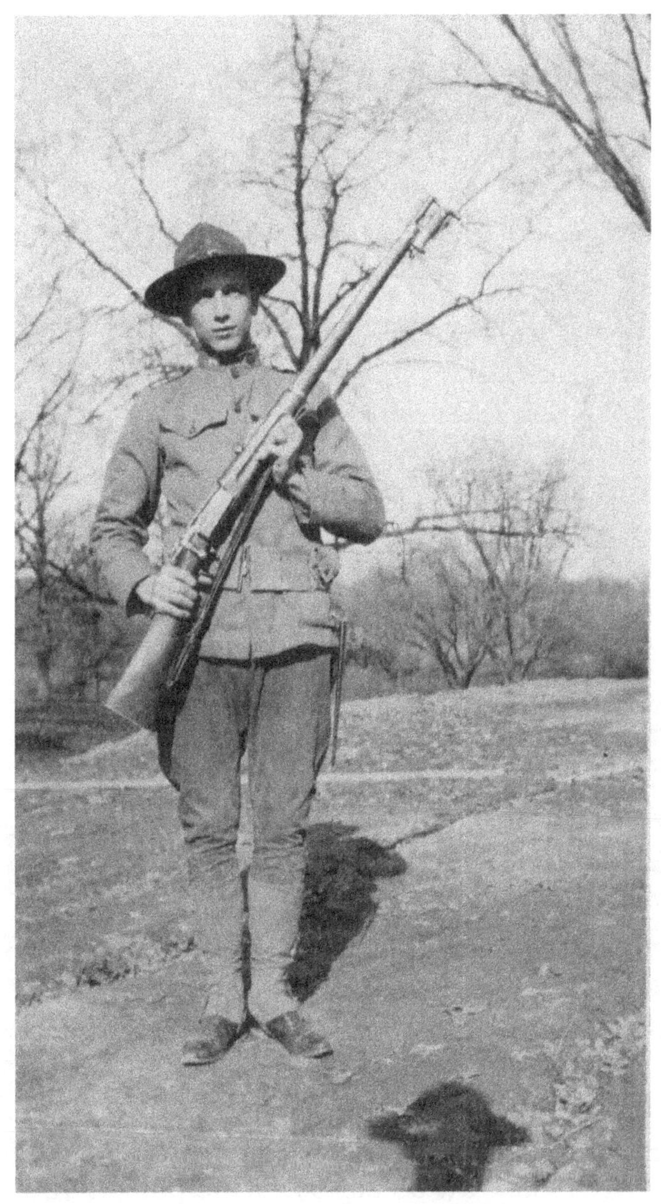

Milo in WW I uniform   November 1918

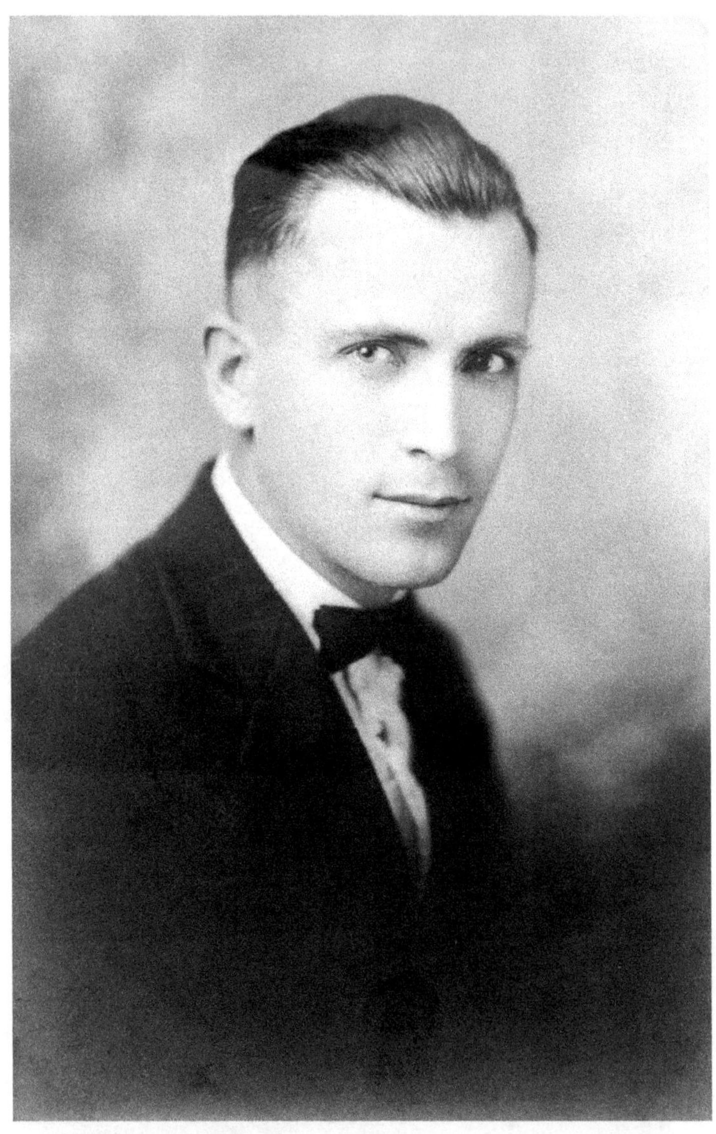

Milo portrait as school principal 1926

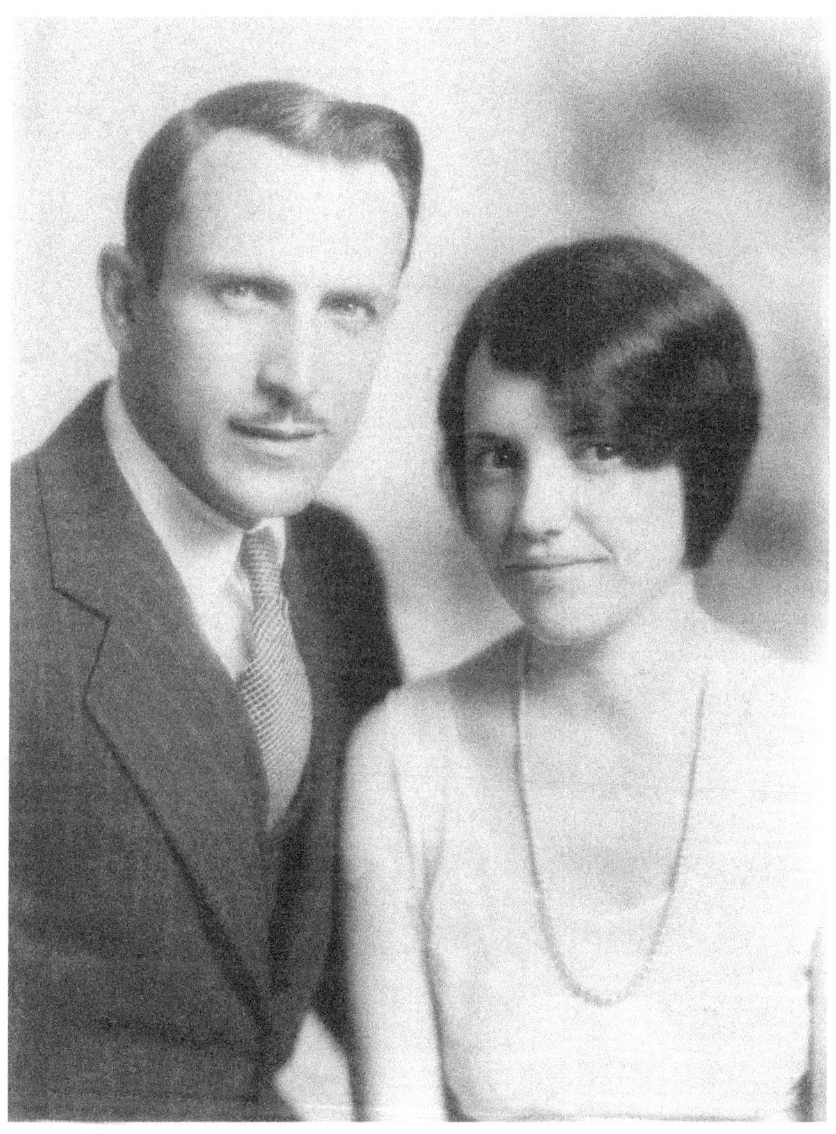

Milo and Eva 1930

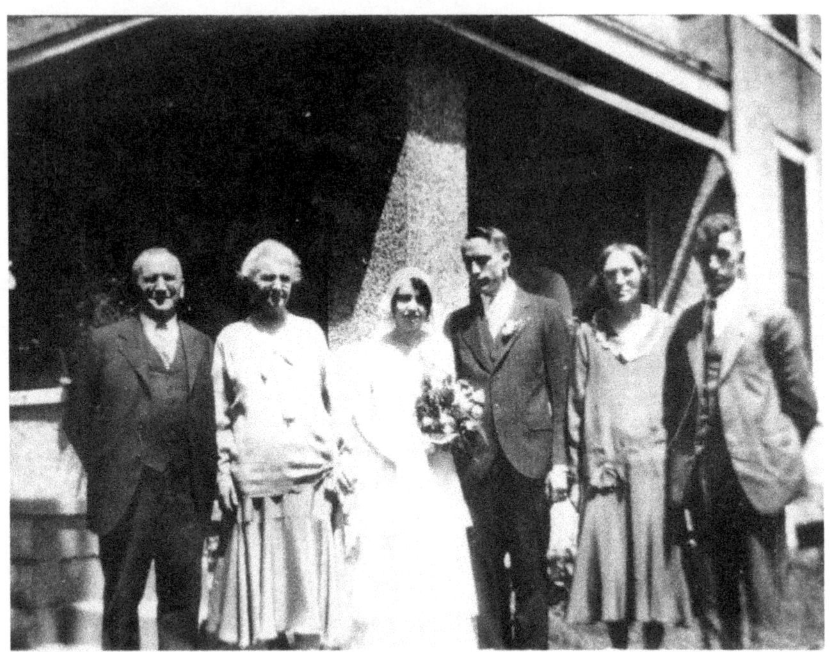

Wedding gathering
Eva's parents, Mr and Mrs. Crawford, Eva and Milo, Melvina and E.E. Brooks

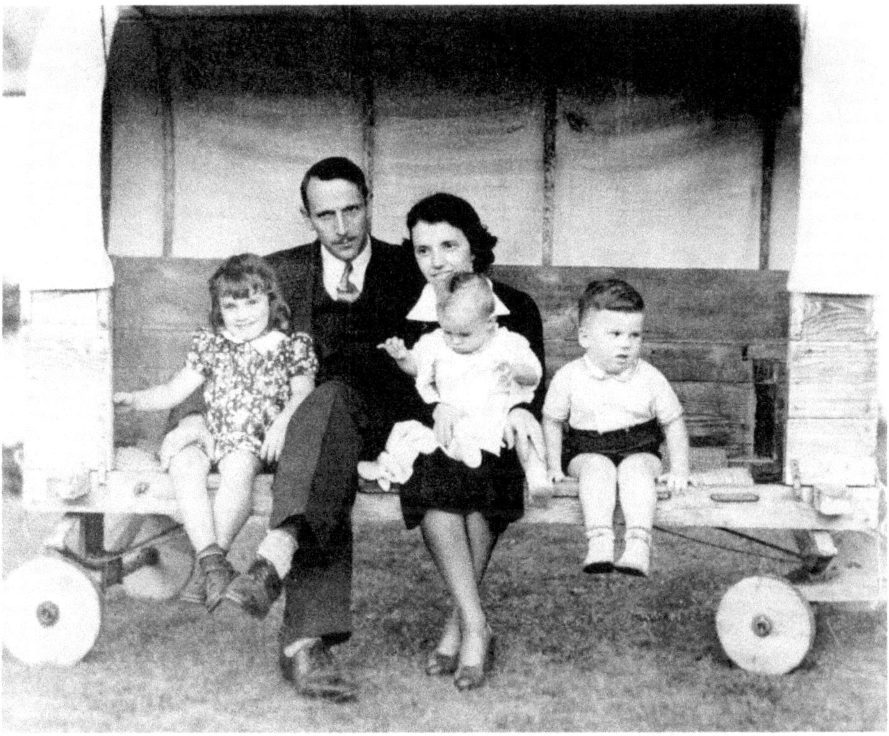

Brooks Family in covered wagon built by Milo 1938
Donna age 5, Ron as a baby, Richard, 3

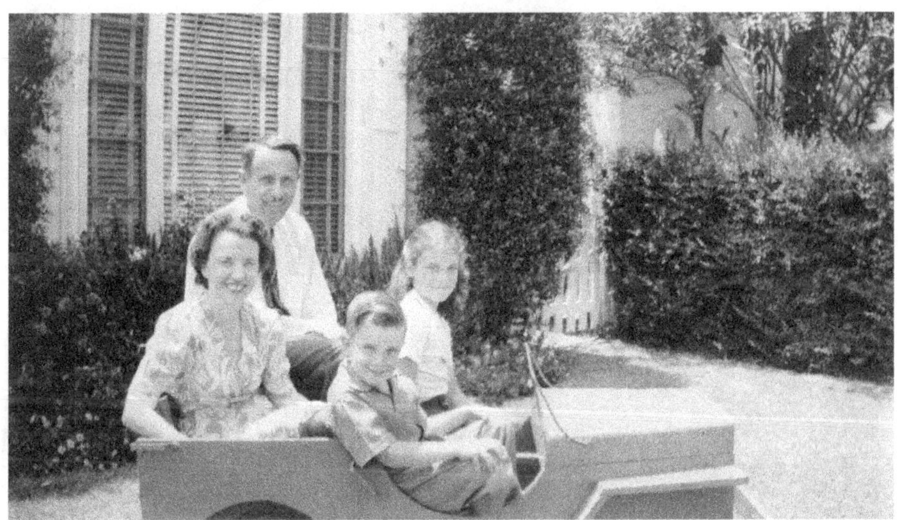

Brooks Family in wooden jeep built by Milo 1943
Donna age 9, Ron age 6

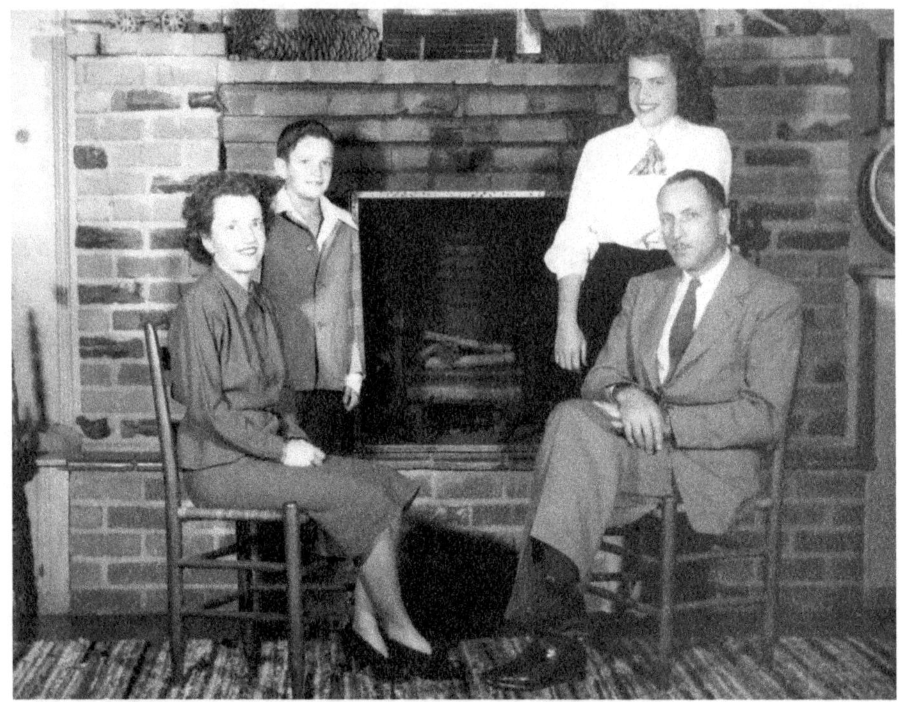

Brooks Family Christmas Card 1950

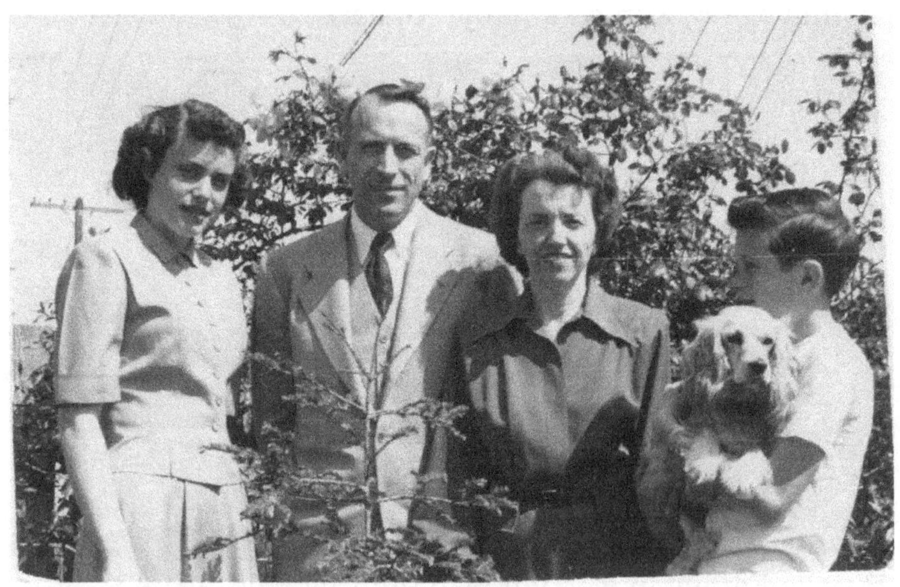

Brooks Family with the baby sequoia tree 1949

FOR THE
LIMB DEFICIENT CHILD

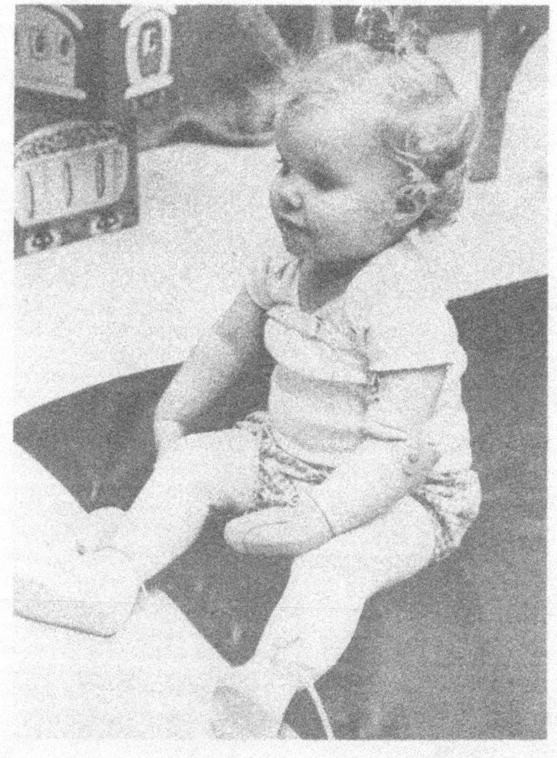

"You handled our boy as if he was a little piece of God."

- A parent.

MILO BROOKS FOUNDATION
for
LIMB DEFICIENT CHILDREN
at the
CHILD AMPUTEE PROSTHETICS PROJECT
UCLA REHABILITATION INSTITUTE

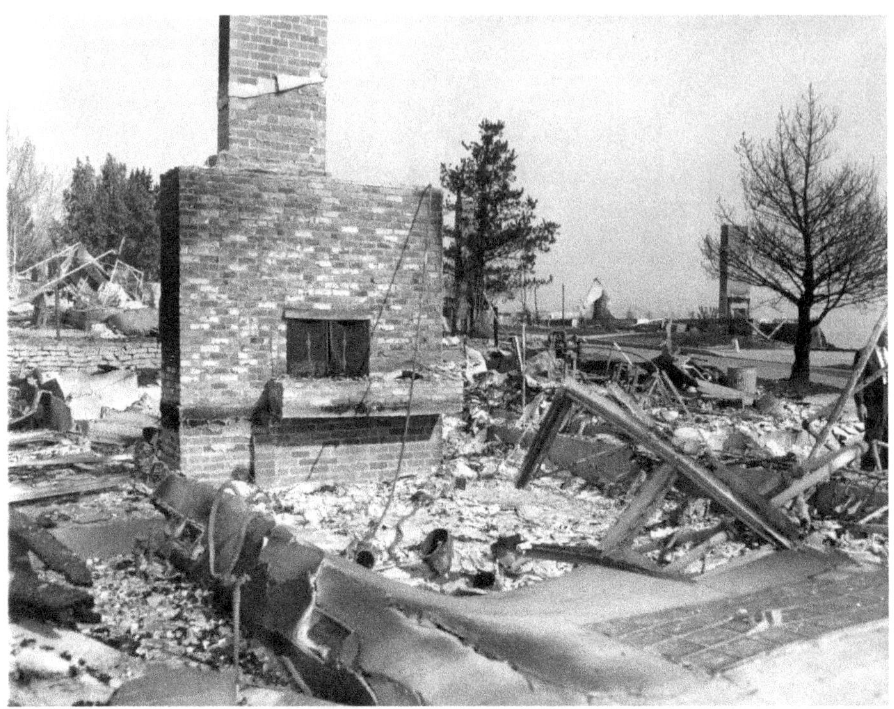

The shell of the house after the fire November, 1961

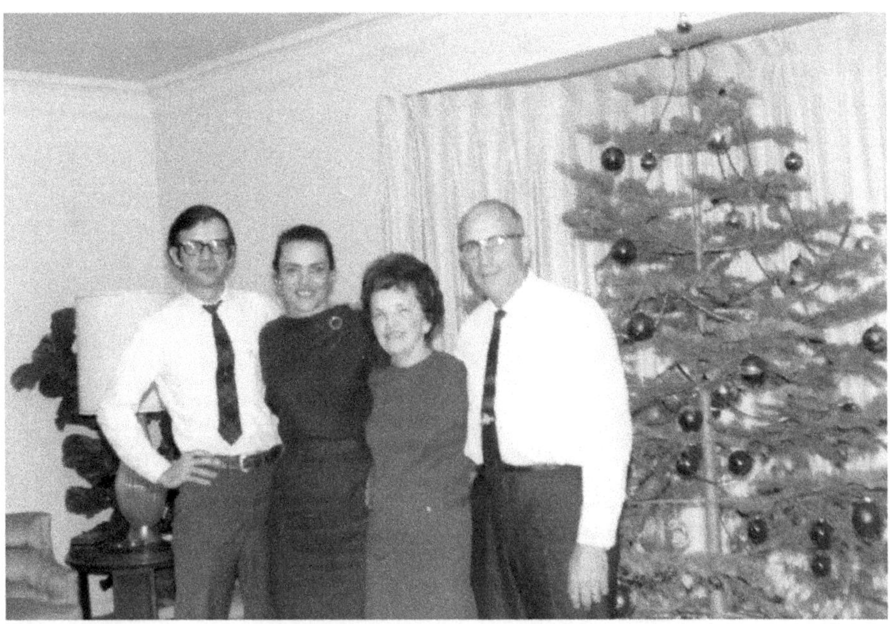

Ron and Donna at home for Christmas, 1967 with their parents

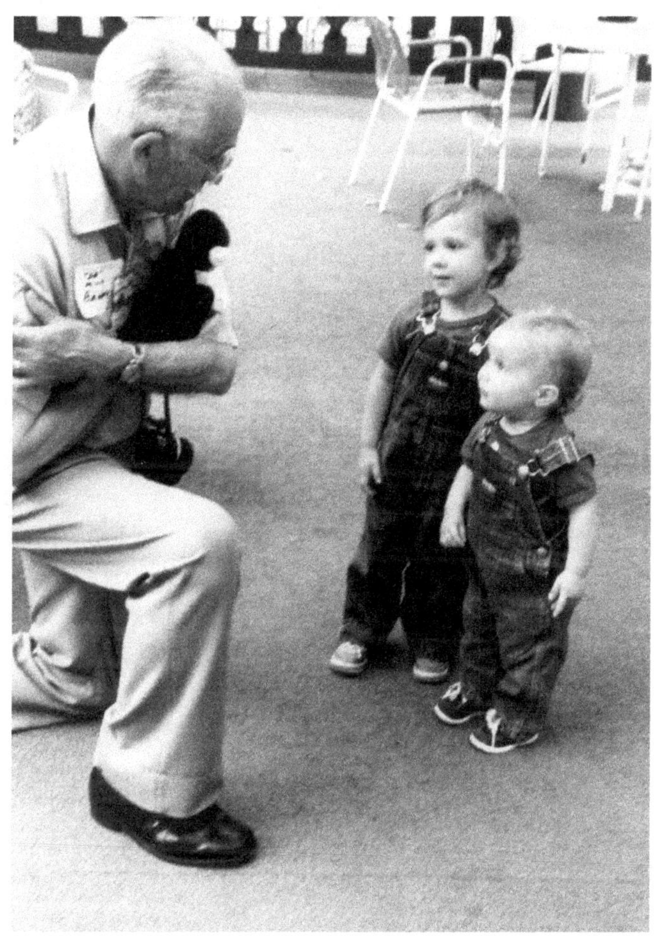

Milo with the hand puppet Bosco and children in 1983

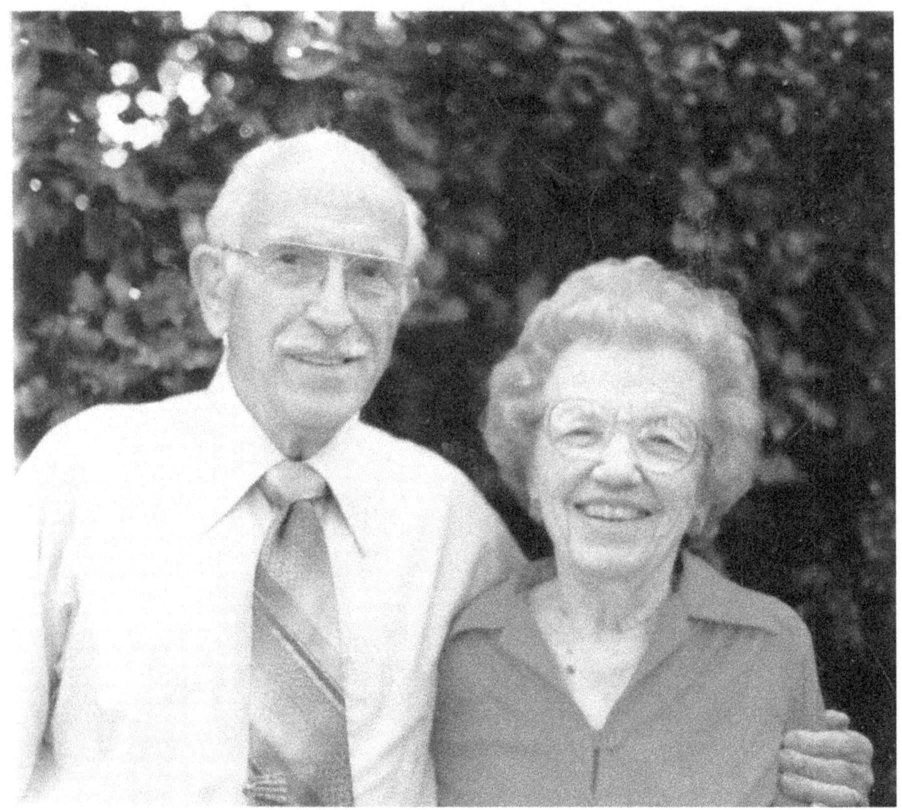

Milo and Eva in 1985

Chapter VI

The Torch is Passed

When Donna Brooks began applying to colleges, she was not thinking of medicine at all; rather she expected to become a physical education teacher. During her years at University High School, she was active in student government and particularly enjoyed a course in leadership. Because she graduated early, in January of 1951, she had several months to fill before the autumn term. First she sold scarves and gloves at a department store. "It was fun," she says, and then she went to work for the librarian at her high school and learned library basics.

Accepted at the University of California at Santa Barbara, Stanford and Pomona College, Donna chose Pomona. When she arrived on campus, the sophomore men greeted the freshmen women and took their measurements. With astonishment she says, "We tolerated it. We were compliant!" Looking back, Donna is now shocked by the learned passivity of her contemporaries. Both Donna and Eva had spent many years thinking that Milo's views and obligations mattered far more than their own and rarely spoke up for their interests. Eva was college educated in an era when very few women were, but she abandoned her career and her music in order to support Milo. Donna was an active member of student representation, and her class of 1955. Some of the members of that class still gather (2013) at Donna's home to laugh and challenge each other's memories.

Pomona was the founding institution of the Claremont Colleges, and has long been known for the passionate loyalty of its graduates. With small class sizes and an atmosphere of engagement in the community, the college maintains to this day its reputation for excellence in teaching which

Donna found so inspiring. Donna enjoyed playing bridge, and if she could not find partners, would teach three people to play. She worked in the dining hall to supplement her funds.

Milo and Eva had at this point never traveled, but decided that Donna should have that opportunity so told her to choose where she wished to go for the six weeks between freshman and sophomore years. She quickly added a Western Civilization course to her studies so that "I would know something of what I was seeing." She flew across the country and then the five-day ocean crossing to Southampton gave her a chance to get to know some of the other students. The group bicycled through southern England and France, took trains through the Alps into Italy, and thoroughly enjoyed their adventures. Eva and Milo were so thrilled by Donna's reports that they began to travel themselves.

A year later Donna was elected as the representative for women students, but to her surprise, the Dean did not allow her to take up the position because she was now a married woman. Between her junior and senior year Donna married a fellow student who was a year ahead of her, a Navy man who was soon deployed abroad. They were divorced after three years, having spent more time apart than together.

The high standard of teaching was not satisfying in her chosen field, and Donna urged the Dean to drop the program in physical education. However, her love of problem solving and her attraction to the sciences led her to apply to the program in physical therapy being taught at the University of Southern California. Her brother Ron was now at the University of California at Santa Barbara, and Donna was concerned about the financial burden on her parents and made a point of financial independence, winning a scholarship to study. The Division of Physical Therapy and Kinesiology was founded at USC in 1945 and is today ranked number one in the nation. Donna found the program well-taught and developed a real passion for anatomy, doing dissection on a cadaver and pursuing a rigorous understanding of the human body.

Milo's responsibility for the prosthetics work was growing, and he was now medical director of the amputee project, but there is no mention in his memoirs of Donna's entry to medicine. As soon as she completed her training, Donna was hired at Rancho Los Amigos National Rehabilitation Center where she was to work for the next several years. Today she puzzles that her professional work did not intersect with Milo's who consulted at Rancho and was friendly with the orthopedists, Dr. Vernon L. Nickel and Dr. Jacqueline Perry. The children's orthopedic service which fused spines and worked with many spinal cord injury and polio patients meant that there were always children rushing about on their "Flexi Flyers", wheeled boards that kept their spines stable, but let them move around the clinics. Sometimes Milo's extensive professional contacts seemed personally intrusive to Donna, but this may have been because he saw himself still in the parental role and not yet as a professional colleague.

Often, visiting Brooks family members came to California; there is a faded Polaroid picture of Julia Brooks visiting Donna at her home in Downey, near Rancho Los Amigos. Donna was now a contributor to the *Brooks Babbler.* With two other physical therapists, Donna returned to Paris for a conference and then visited more places than she had toured earlier. One Christmas when Eva and Milo came to her home, Donna brought one of the paralyzed polio patients to share the festivities. She rented an ambulance, supplied the respirator, and helped the patient taste all aspects of the dinner. This incident shows an aspect of her caring for the person, not merely the disease, which would become even more frequent when she became a physician.

It was very unusual at the time that one of the leading orthopedists at Rancho was a woman. As Donna became aware that she could do more as a physician than as a physical therapist, she thought perhaps she could pursue a career in orthopedics. First, however, she had to complete the prerequisites for medical school, and then, as a mature student, she had to find a medical school that would accept her for study. She was able to finish her chemistry, physics, mathematics and foreign language requirements in Long Beach. Only seven per cent of physicians were women at this time, and there was a strong bias toward taking only students younger than age twenty-five. Each medical school had different admission requirements, so it was hard to anticipate what might be required.

The Women's Medical College of Pennsylvania opened in 1850, and was the only medical college founded for women studying to become physicians. Donna had never heard of it at the time she applied, but quickly learned that they were strong advocates of nontraditional students, believing that those with more life experience had more to offer as physicians. When they accepted Donna to study beginning in the autumn of 1961, and gave her a scholarship, little did they know that she would be an eager advocate for their exceptional history and tradition and an active participant in the evolution of the institution. The history of women's medical education has been written elsewhere but it is worth noting that Harvard did not admit women until 1945, almost a century after the founding of the Philadelphia college.

At the Women's Medical College of Pennsylvania all members of the faculty were boarded in their particular specialty, and Donna found them passionate about teaching. The model was very much an apprenticeship system, with each teacher getting to know the student as a person, and letting the students know them. Looking back on this remarkable education from the year 2000, Donna was concerned about the changes happening to her school, and sponsored "Essays of a Legacy, Portraits of Women Physicians" by River Malcolm. These are interviews with the retiring mentors who, in Donna's words "made the school what it was".

The WMCP environment was deeply humane, and when the history of its Quaker traditions influenced the student, they became the guardians and stewards of a sacred trust on behalf of women. Donna was especially impressed that learning was collaborative and cooperative, not competitive. At first she roomed with two other students, but she found that the contrasting habits bothered her study, and even after changing her sleep so that she got up to study at two in the morning, the situation was frustrating. Later, when Donna was the senior resident, she worked very hard at the schedule to be sure all assignments were fair, but another student ripped up the schedule that had taken Donna so many hours to complete. "Not everyone was cooperative," she says.

Early in her studies, Donna was disappointed in her grades, and Milo wrote:

> *"Don't give up yet, or ever.*
>
> *"I firmly believe that every disappointment can be used to some good advantage."*

One of the important aspects of training, and of the culture at WMCP, was that the physician was to be 'hands-on'. Palpation taught the physician so much that mechanical monitoring misses. Further, it enhanced the trust and intimacy between the physician and the patient which significantly contributed to healing. Donna maintains today that every physician needs to know how to do a hands-on history and physical diagnosis of the patient—"that is the craft, the art, the joy that makes medicine healing." If all the tools and technologies create dependence on the part of the physician, what will happen when the electricity fails? Or when you need to know more than machines can tell you? Just as Milo had placed mirrors behind his examination table to watch how carefully he was handling infants and children, Donna continued the vigilant art.

When asked, Milo denied that he was an influence in Donna's choice of medicine, and Donna herself does not believe that he was, yet there are commonalities and resonant themes that become ever more obvious as Donna worked to become a physician. Donna says that Milo's admonition was no matter what she chose to do she should give that choice her best effort. He also said that the most important thing about being a physician was that "the nurses must like you".

Shortly after her enrollment in Philadelphia, the fire destroyed Milo and Eva's home, and Donna returned briefly to assure herself that her parents were well. There is only one mention in Milo's Memoirs of Donna's years in medical school:

> *Dr. Waldo Nelson was also my guest in Los Angeles when he came to address pediatric meetings; we became friends and he later invited me to speak at Children's Hospital in Philadelphia, which I did on the day President Kennedy was shot. Our daughter, Donna was in medical school in Philadelphia at the time and helped by running the film and slides for my talk. Also that day I met C. Everett Koop who is now in 1982 the Surgeon General of the U.S.*

But in some editions of the *Babbler* there are more details.

> *Donna has finished her Junior year and will be starting Senior next week. On August 2nd she starts a six week externship at Los Angeles County Harbor General Hospital in Torrance [California] and then will have four weeks' vacation until about October tenth. She will then go back to Philadelphia and graduate in June 1965.*

During this 'vacation' Donna taught anatomy at Rancho Los Amigos. Returning to Philadelphia, Donna had to choose an internship and begin to think of a specialty.

The orthopedics department at Women's Medical College was not as large or as varied as the obstetrics and gynecology department, and primarily specialized in microscopic work which did not interest Donna. But first came graduation, of importance to the large Brooks clan.

> *Donna won the department award for work in Obstetrics and Gynecology besides the Honorary AOA Society.*

She was accepted to the intern class at Harbor General Hospital in Los Angeles, associated with UCLA, with thirty other students. The only other woman dropped out before the end of the year. Donna had been aware in Philadelphia that many of the women were never sure of their standing, and needed reassurance from older practitioners, but quickly as an intern Donna was aware that her training had been at least as good, and more often better, than that of her male colleagues. Harbor General Hospital was a new hospital, with new equipment, and the interns were given a great deal of responsibility.

Just as in the years in Philadelphia, the intern year was demanding and concentrated. Reviewing Donna's surgical notes from her Intern year, which along with many other records, she has preserved, the reader is struck by how cogent they are. Frequently Donna would correct grammar and spelling in the notes made by others, and she was careful to be sure that reference was made to the person's overall health. When she would later be in the operating room, she admonished her assistants to remember that the patient could hear and remember what was said around them.

As a medical student, Donna had joined her peers bowling on Wednesday afternoons, but she had no time to get to know Philadelphia or to have any real relaxation. Now she seemed to have no time off, and Milo and Eva complained that they saw her too rarely. Around her birthday in 1965, they held a party and invited seventy-five people.

Milo reported to the family:

> *Donna has accepted a four year Residency in Obstetrics and Gynecology at Women's Medical College in Philadelphia beginning in July 1966. It is a good opportunity to get started in medical school teaching if she desires. She is on Pediatrics Service now and I am technically on the staff at Harbor Hospital, so hope to make rounds with her some time.*

Milo was concerned for the demands upon his daughter:

> *Donna has some long, hard days. On her two months of OB service she delivered over one hundred babies and now is on General Surgery.*

Milo and Eva were now traveling extensively, but tried to stop in Philadelphia as often as possible. They spent Christmas of 1968 with Donna. Milo writes in the *Babbler*:

> *I was able to watch Donna deliver a baby boy by Caesarian Section on Christmas Day. She wields a knife and sutures with expertise.*

At the end of August 1969, Milo and Eva tell the family:

> *Donna is home and has passed her Obstetrics and Gynecology Board examinations. She has been looking for a place to practice in Southern California.*

Life was busy and changing for all of the Brooks family, but again, it is Rena who comments on the world beyond family and professional concerns:

> *That moon landing was exciting. I sat here between the two big windows that evening watching them and could look out the window to my left and see the big bright moon in the sky while seeing them walk on it. Fantastic. Such perfect timing and operation of it all.*

Milo and Eva urged Donna to take up practice in Santa Monica, which would be near them, but she liked San Diego and explored opportunities there. First, however, she accepted a *locum tenens* position in Downey. She arrived on a Friday hoping for the list from the doctor as to who was in the hospital and what she might expect. Instead, the doctor said she was leaving for Australia that afternoon and would be back in a month.

Wryly, Donna remembers:

> *I cannot have inspired much confidence showing up at a hospital and asking 'Where's Labor and Delivery?'*

Milo kept up somehow and reported to the family:

> *It's a very busy experience. Eight deliveries and one Caesarean the first week besides office every day except Sunday.*

The demand for women doctors by women was increasing, and in San Diego, Donna joined the practice of another female OB/Gyn so that they could share call. They were delivering babies all over San Diego County at the several hospitals and were able to keep up with the demand. Then Donna encountered a patient of the other doctor who said she had been 'promised' that she would not have any IV during her delivery. Much as Milo had eventually refused to accept patients who refused immunizations, Donna felt that such a promise compromised patient care, as the physician must be able to decide what to do if the need arose; recognizing that it was time, she set up her independent practice.

By April of 1970, she had bought a home, and Milo was telling the family that he wanted to go down to San Diego to 'do odd jobs' at the new house. When Milo was away the following spring, Eva wrote the family:

> *I spent a pleasant weekend with Donna in San Diego. Donna's patients were considerate as she only had to deliver two babies while I was there. She was at the hospital until 1:30 on Friday night but otherwise her sleep was not badly interrupted.*

In August of 1972, Milo fell down some cement steps, breaking his ribs; x-rays showed that there were fifteen fractures in all. For the first time, Donna had oversight of his medical care, although she was doing so as a devoted daughter, arranging home visits, instructing him how to move safely, and being sure her mother got some respite. By Christmas time, Milo was well enough to take the grandchildren to Mexico, but he recognized that it had been a serious injury. In April of 1974, when Eva was ill, Donna again was vigilant on her mother's behalf.

In September of 1974, Rena, Milo's older sister died, and writing of his memories of her Milo captures some of the feeling of his memoirs.

> *My earliest recollection of her is when she was ten and shepherding four of us younger ones to school. Back in Iowa at sixteen she was delighted to be nearing her cherished hopes of High School graduation. Then this had to be postponed for teacher training and several years teaching to bring in cash income for the family. Many times her encouragement kept me on the goal for a medical education. Every member of the family of nine reached equal or more education than she had.*

Donna took her parents to a four-day seminar at Pomona College in July of 1975, twenty years after her graduation, and Milo was reflective. The subject of the seminar was "What has happened to the American Dream?" He could see that his life was part of that story. He was still traveling extensively for the prosthetics project, but seeing Donna build her practice was prompting him to reflect more on his own work. By this time, Maurice, now over ninety, and

Milo had started writing their respective memories, and their siblings were eager to read more.

Visits to San Diego, and from San Diego to Westwood were routine, and now Donna was the physician to whom others in the family turned for good advice and loving attention; when Ron was injured or in pain, he now went to someone Donna recommended in San Diego for diagnosis and care. Donna was doing her best to case manage the fragilities of the family, and while Milo was the last person to admit to fragility, it was clear that Donna's skills were appreciated.

Milo reported:

> *Donna was on call and very busy with seven deliveries from Thursday to Monday besides office hours and several scheduled surgeries. I watched a difficult delivery one night and was proud of her expertise and concern for the patient.*

It is clear that Milo could not tell Donna to her face how much he admired her as a physician, but certainly his pride in her is conveyed throughout the *Babbler.* When finally in 1980 Milo began his memoirs, Donna was not only often the typist, but frequently she prompted him to tell more stories of medicine, of his practice, of the changes he had experienced.

Donna recently rediscovered a letter Milo wrote to her as she began medicine:

> *We think we have a mighty fine daughter, Donna. We are proud of you, not just because you are going to be a Doctor nor even in spite of it. It is pride that you have found something you prize highly enough to work as hard as you will have to. You have a background that will make you one of the finest Doctors. Love, Dad*

Milo and Eva travelled often, frequently with Donna and her second husband Mort Weisman (an anesthesiologist).

Milo was still receiving awards at various conferences, but he comments that he has to rest more often and does not have the energy often to do, or to eat, what was offered.

The profession entered fifty years before, and the tradition of the closely knit homesteading community, would continue. The torch had been passed.

Chapter VII

To See the Patient as Whole

Throughout the Seventies Donna was extremely busy, building her practice, fulfilling professional obligations, and mentoring student doctors. In the early months, when she had the time, she volunteered at the University of California San Diego free clinics, which continued until UCSD had its own faculty. Soon however, she was in demand with a seven-month waiting list at one point, except for physician referral.

Educating the patients about what was happening in their bodies and what she was doing was vitally important to Donna. She wanted the women she treated to understand, so that together they could work not only for the specific desired outcome of treatment, but better health. Many of her patients seemed unable to remember which 'pill' they were on, so Donna created a bulletin board with samples of over thirty different contraceptive pills, and ("usually") the patient could identify the package. Some drug representatives wanted to copy Donna's innovation, she recalls, but she does not know if they ever did.

One day, when she was President of the San Diego Gynecological Society, she herself was scheduled for a CAT scan and knew she was allergic to the dye which was used. Despite premedication, she began to have shortness of breath in the radiology department, which was not used to handling emergencies. The department called a Code Blue when Donna's distress escalated. That evening she showed up to the Society's commemorative dinner, somewhat subdued, but she says, she was still able to introduce the speakers! This is reminiscent of Milo's Rotary motto: Service Above Self.

She was expansive and inclusive in her approach to women's health and persuaded Sharp Hospital in San Diego to help her offer gynecological services to women with disabilities and to those suffering from various levels of paralysis. She established the protocols for gynecological care of these women. Women in wheelchairs were rarely examined outside the chairs, so Donna found ways to apply her skills on their behalf. She was never paid for these services, offering her expertise because it was needed, as Milo had resolved to do in his practice.

As Donna's reputation spread, she was often called for problematic situations. Not only was she asked to write the protocol for the evaluation of rape victims, but Children's Hospital called her to help an infant who had been raped with a pencil and was bleeding internally. She and the surgical nurse had to figure out what instruments were small enough to be of use as Donna treated the injury. They had to use a nasal speculum for the infant vagina.

What was the state of primary care for women during this time? Let us think of Donna's grandmother, Melvina, who bore ten children, raised nine of them to adulthood and lived from the homesteading era to the post-WWII era without much recourse to professional medicine. In part that may have been due to her religious beliefs, but it was also due to the assumptions of the day: childbirth was a normal event, it was not seen as requiring hospital care; most maladies could be handled by a woman, with the help of experienced neighbors, on behalf of her family, and physicians were useful for emergencies and infectious diseases, but not for much else. Death and pain were accepted as reality, not as enemies, and living was activity engaged with and for other people. There were moments of agony in life, but they were to be endured; no prescription was sought for what was viewed as the human condition. The scientific understanding of human reproduction had been established in 1843, and the contraceptive pill was approved for use in 1960; this was the century of Melvina Brooks' life. Hygiene became the source of public protection from infection; we remember that Milo got in trouble at school for tracing the route of the lice dropping from the hair of the girl in front of him. Technology beyond the stethoscope and x-rays was introduced slowly; and these two were the basic tools available for diagnosis. Donna practiced as the technological revolution took place.

Nevertheless, fraudulent and dangerous offerings were advertised, First Lady Eleanor Roosevelt took the "America's Chamber of Horrors Exhibit" to the White House to advocate for strong protections for women. Among the exhibits was a weight-loss drug that caused death, a hair remover that caused baldness and lotions that could cause mercury or lead poisoning. It was not until 1962 that the Kefauver-Harris Amendments to the Food, Drug and Cosmetic Act of 1938 required that drugs be proven effective before being marketed.

In Donna's letters to her parents, while they were in Europe learning about Thalidomide, she comments that it would be a very good thing if medicines had to be approved as safe and effective before they could be marketed. The huge controlled study of the Salk polio vaccine from 1953 to 1955 was then, and still remains, unique in its scope regarding safety and proof of efficacy.

"I loved the practice of medicine," says Donna. She is an artist, and she means practice in the same way that a great pianist would refer to practice. She was dedicated to constant improvement of her skills, and curious about innovations and experiments that could lead to improved ways for dealing with physical challenges. If you ask her to recall some surgical or clinical drama or challenge, she smiles and says

> *Surgeons do not think that way, we think of the problem to be solved which is before us, it is something to be dealt with, that's all.*

Similarly, if you ask her to remember the first time she operated, or did a particular procedure, her modesty sets the tone:

> *As soon as the retractors are in place for abdominal surgery, you cannot tell whose hands are doing something first, there is no single control. In an experienced team, you work together, always and in all ways, whether you are the surgeon of record or the assistant. This is not the case always, or with an experienced surgeon and students.*

In the spring of 1973, Donna moved into her own office; Eva described it:

> *It is in the same building but needs to be redecorated, have some new cabinets put in etc. Of course Milo was eager to see what he could do to help. Three doctors in the other office were quite crowded and there was no extra space near them. Donna's office will have four examine rooms, two rooms for the secretaries and records, a small lab, her consultation room, and a good size reception room.*

Milo reflected after the move "now she will have to work hard."

Working hard and long and relentlessly on behalf of others was Donna's nature, just as it was Milo's. She had not chosen academic medicine, but she mentored many young physicians and constantly tried to refer patients to women who were starting out in practice. Women were now eager to have female OB-Gyn physicians. One of her mentees, or students, is Barbara Levy, who is now the Vice-President for Health Policy for the American College of Obstetricians and Gynecologists. Donna remembers one of their days together:

> *I was in my jeans going to a pharmacy on the weekend. There was a woman sitting on a bench*

> *outside, clearly she was in pain. I asked if I could help and she said she was getting pain medication from the pharmacist. So I asked more questions and began to suspect that she had an ectopic pregnancy. She said her aunt was waiting for her in the car, so I told them to meet me at the closest hospital, which was Mission Bay. We went to the Emergency Room and established that she did have a ruptured ectopic pregnancy. When I operated, I found she had a belly full of blood. Ever afterward, Barb Levy teased me that I could not go alone to a pharmacy, or I would "pick-up" patients.*

The laughter is typical of the self-deprecation in Donna's attitude toward her skills. She had just intervened and saved a life, but it was the teasing that makes her laugh. Medicine was changing significantly in these years. Patients wanted more information, asked more questions, and were interested in natural childbirth. Patients were still compliant with the physician's advice, but wanted to take a more active role in their own prenatal care.

Electronic Uterine Monitoring of the fetal heartbeat was introduced in the 1970s, as was the use of ultrasound. Epidurals were becoming much more common during labor and delivery, and laparoscopy was first developed by gynecologists, who then taught the skills required for it to other surgeons. Donna was concerned not only about the broad applications of new technology, but about the intrusion of technology between the patient and the physician. She was on the clinical teaching faculty at Mercy Hospital in San Diego, and for the University of California at San Diego Medical School, and she was profoundly aware that the skills of a physician might diminish if they relied on sources of information external to their observation and rapport with the patient. No young physician was allowed to scrub in with Donna unless they had first done a hands-on history and physical examination of the patient.

Donna was concerned when husbands began to demand that they be present in the operating room during a Caesarean section delivery. "A surgeon's attention must not be divided," she comments. In the ordinary delivery room, she was amused that frequently husbands maintained that their wives needed 'no pain medication.'

The River Malcolm book on WMCP physicians quotes Donna about surgery:

> *Donna Brooks once compared surgery to the creative process of an artist; just as an artist may discover that her painting or book evolves into something very different from what she expected, so the surgeon can be taken by surprise by the actual body of the patient. Asked if she ever worried about what she would find, or was frightened by what she did find, Donna replied, "I'm always intensely curious at what each body will be like. No two are exactly the same. It is forever interesting and a challenge. You have to make decisions in the moment—with all the planning you can do—the moment of entry into the body is always a moment of great and sacred mystery.*

Essays of a Legacy, P. 58

Gradually, Donna recognized that she could not be up all night with a delivery, and then be fresh for surgery in the morning. She changed her focus to surgery and gynecology so that she no longer dealt with the demands of labor and delivery. Milo's admonition that the nurses must like her was somewhat ironic, in that Donna inspired a remarkable loyalty and trust in all who worked with her and all who were cared for by her. Whenever she herself became a patient, nurses argued over who would have the 'privilege' of caring for her. More than twenty years after her retirement, one of her office nurses still comes to San Diego from Atlanta to visit.

In 1984, Donna was honored by the San Diego YWCA "Tribute to Women and Industry" program. Richard L. Keyser was president of Mercy Hospital and commented:

> *Dr. Brooks is a mentor and role model for many young women considering a career in medicine. She is known as a model physician with very high professional standards.*
>
> *Her involvement in medical/political/academic organizations is extensive. Dr. Brooks has served as President of the San Diego Gyn Society, and as a Vice President of the San Diego and Orange Counties section of the American College of OB-Gyn, to name but two of her many accomplishments.*

Once more we hear an echo of Milo Brooks who was repeatedly honored for his contributions to his profession and to clinical medicine. Yet, let us not forget Eva, for much of the self-effacing service that characterizes Donna's life is resonant of Eva and her role, as it is of the courage of Melvina, her grandmother, who urged everyone to "Learn patience and be understanding."

Three major changes in medicine would tax Donna's patience and challenge her confidence in where her profession was going. These were the explosion of malpractice insurance and changes in those laws; the intrusion of insurance companies into clinical decision-making, and the direct marketing of drugs and procedures to patients. Various technologies had greatly increased therapeutic distancing. These have taken the physician's attention from the words—the narrative—of the patient to a particular aspect of reality, measured or amplified by the technical tool. If this partial reality of data is compelling so that the physician can call it 'evidence', then it may become a substitute for the whole, which is a far more complex reality. Donna was, and is, profoundly committed to the sacred trust given to the physician, and to the mystery that is both the body, and the person. In the 1970s physicians were being held accountable in law for bad outcomes, whether or not their skills had anything to do with those outcomes.

One of the attractions that obstetrics provided for Donna was the reality that the physician must have a wide variety of skills to deal with the issues that even a healthy pregnancy involves, and thus, the physician is more profoundly involved in caring for the mother and baby. The explosion of malpractice costs also came with the 'long tail' of risk, which meant that the delivering physician could be sued until the infant reached the age of twenty-one. As Donna commented

> *It does not help your focus as you meet someone in the examining room, or enter the operating theater, if you worry that they might sue you at any time in the next twenty-one years.*

In the years since her retirement, many areas of the nation have found that women have inadequate access to obstetricians because so few are willing to practice with this burden upon them. Given the economics, the only way to meet the financial burden would have been to see more patients for a shorter amount of time, or in Donna's view, to compromise the quality of care, or to practice in a group and share the cost of the overhead. However, with the introductions of managed care, both hospitals and insurance companies were demanding just this kind of approach. In addition, as the fragmented diagnostic technologies measured minute incidents, symptoms and mechanisms, the physician's role changed from being one who cares for and educates another person, to one who fixes a part or repairs damage. This diminishes both the transformative role of the physician and the narrative reporting by the patient. Donna reflects: "The relationship between the physician and her patient has to be based on empathy; it cannot be a contest, and it cannot be based on mutual fear."

Insurance systems often act as if the management of risk by both the physician and the patient must be based upon fear, and this too demeans the trust necessary to healing. We recall the poem praising Milo's lesson in loving the limb deficient baby. Without trust, such lessons can neither be learned nor taught. Many insurance companies attempt to manage risk—and increase profit—by restricting what the physician may and may not do, so that reimbursement rather than trust drives the application of medical skills. This takes away the art, and the craft, from medicine in the view of many physicians. "Medicine cannot be joyous" under these circumstances says Donna.

As she was facing these dilemmas, Donna was at the top of her profession. Several landlords tried to recruit her to locate in a particular building. Finally one group persuaded her with the promise that the office could be built to her design. Donna the artist found a real outlet in instituting many ideas ranging from the warm and comfortable color scheme to using warm wraps called ruannas, instead of little paper exam gowns, installing a washer and dryer in the back office and having real art grace the walls. In 1988, this office opened, and the practice was now limited to gynecology.

Donna wrote in the *Babbler* that

> *the fresh new environment is invigorating.*

When former patients visit to share their stories and appreciation of Donna's care, they often speak of the laughter in the office, and the sense of delight Donna conveyed in seeing them and caring for them.

These were busy and yet often sad years. Both Ron and Milo died, and Eva's capacities were increasingly limited, although she enjoyed music and concerts when possible. Donna and Mort had been divorced, and by the late eighties, Donna began to experience the sudden pain and 'flare-ups' that would be diagnosed as rheumatoid arthritis. Frequently she was visited by WMCP friends, and often her travels were to meet them and participate in medical conferences. It is remarkable that each time the *Brooks Babbler* was sent on by Donna to the rest of the family, she made a personal comment on everyone's news and made sure they each knew that she felt connected to them. Donna feels deeply obligated to the family and the tradition she has inherited. She is always especially warm in her remarks on Ron's two children and the others of the next generation. When a cousin is hospitalized, or when another reports a success, Donna promptly writes to clarify and to comfort and to encourage.

When Donna worried that flares of rheumatoid pain might occur during surgery, she knew it was time to retire. In September of 1991 she performed her final operation and closed her practice. Typically, she donated the furniture to a women's shelter, and the equipment to the hospital. Donna's letter to her patients is a lesson in the true meaning of good medicine in every sense:

> *It is with mixed feelings that I write to tell you of my decision to retire and close my practice at the end of this September 1991. As you know, medicine has been a part of my entire life. It has been a richly rewarding experience to form such special associations with both my patients and my colleagues. I have had the extraordinary privilege to be with many of you at the moment of the miracle of birth. I have delighted in watching the children that I delivered and their mothers grow and mature. And since giving up the 'night life' of obstetrics seven years ago, I have enjoyed shepherding many into the 'golden years'. Surgery has been a special love of mine throughout. It has meant a great deal to be such a trusted part of your lives in both sickness and health. Few people in the world are allowed such an intimate sharing of people's lives; for this I thank you all. I will miss this part of my life greatly. I hope you will keep in touch with me through the years as you have in the past.*

> *I have become increasingly aware of the time and energy demands that the practice of medicine imposes. There is no way that one can do it well, keeping up with the rapid advances in medicine, without it being an all encompassing obligation. I do not know how to practice medicine part time.*

There are two volumes of appreciative letters from patients and colleagues written at the time of her retirement. A simple chronology of service at only one hospital is an astonishing testament to her service:

October 1969 joined the medical staff

Tissue Committee 1976

Medical Record Committee 1977

Risk Management

OB-Gyn Supervisory Committee 1976-1991

Blood Transfusion 1981

Credentials Committee 1984-1990

Women's Program Advisory Board

Impaired Physician's Committee

She served equally diligently at five other hospitals and constantly mentored young women entering her profession. One such wrote upon receiving notice of her retirement:

> *Dear Donna*
>
> *It is with confused emotions that I write to you as both a colleague and a patient, to respond to your upcoming retirement.*
>
> *I am very happy for you, knowing that you are a very creative person and will now have the time to*

> *pursue other interests. However, I am already becoming nostalgic looking back at our relationship and what a beautiful role model you have been for me. Your support 'through thick and thin' will always be remembered and appreciated. I have to say that you are truly a courageous woman, not only for playing a 'pioneer' role for women in medicine, but also for recognizing the time for self-fulfillment.*
>
> *Nancy S. Cetel, M.D.*

Other physicians wrote thanking Donna for the referrals that helped them start their practices and, repeatedly, for being a role model for women. Another surgeon comments:

> *I am quite sympathetic to the problem of trying to find enough time in the day to live like a human being and continue the sole practice of medicine. I wish you well in your endeavor to continue growth and development without the burden of daily demands from your medical practice.*
>
> *Richard M. Braun, M.D.*

Another physician wrote:

> *It has been a great pleasure for me to have labored in the vineyard with you these many years. Your name has been a symbol of excellence and kindness; a true practitioner of the art of medicine.*
>
> *John J. Stevens, MD*

For Donna, as for Milo, the humanity of medicine, the sacred trust, commanded total dedication, at the expense of many other aspects of living.

One of the best summations of Donna's dedication is by River Malcolm, the poet:

Her Hands

They have reached deeply
into the innermost mysteries of the flesh
unflinchingly cut through living skin and bone,
moved muscles, loosened ligaments,
and calmed the storming panic of the blood.

They have reached deep
inside the mysteries of life
Inside the temple of the god, of flesh,
the great replenisher.
These hands have held and bent life
to their dreams, and bid flesh mend
along their careful seams.

These hands have spanned
as few have ever done
both intellect's precise technology—
that views in icy light
the body's most impersonal geometry
and so manipulates, with gestures
sure, detached, and right—
and heart's astonished reverence—
whose subtle fingers meet
and are transformed by
each rare soul embodied in a flesh uniquely
strange, a flake of human snow, no two alike.

These hands have suffered, and may suffer more
a crippling pain, the flesh god's shadow side.
lifelong, they strive to limit and contain
the shadow of their god:
These hands know well
that flesh, the great replenisher,
is also mother of decay.
As healer and as sufferer, these hands
do wrestle with the god they love.
These hands do wrestle with the god of life.

River Malcolm, September 27, 1991

It was, and still is, a source of great sorrow to Donna that she could not find a physician who would take over her practice and patients and treat them with similar dedication and care.

> *Everyone I interviewed only wanted to know how much money they would make and what hours they would work, so it seemed better to close the doors rather than compromise the quality. I searched for a long time, but failed to find anyone.*

After a grand retirement party, generously arranged by Cathy Conheim, Donna's partner, others perhaps thought that Donna's life would be distant from medicine. Instead, Donna translated her skills from professional services to advocacy and began to use her healing hands in a new and very different way.

Patients who had no family support frequently recuperated at Donna and Cathy's home, and were repeatedly, after abdominal surgery, admonished by Donna to "Stand up straight.' Some would stay as long as two weeks, feeling safer as long as Donna was present. Patients who were afraid of a surgery sometimes found Donna beside them in the operating room, and certainly during recovery. She, better than anyone else, could explain what was happening and share her serenity as part of their healing. During particularly severe flu seasons, Donna would obtain the vaccine and be sure that those who would not otherwise get the immunization did so. Some Thanksgiving dinners were especially funny, as between the turkey and the dessert, twenty or more guests would line up for their shots.

One woman suffered for years from a wound that would not heal, and Donna shepherded her through that long course of treatment. Sometimes a child of a frail parent would call from across the country and ask Donna to determine what was going on; at other times, colleagues would ask for her intervention. Whatever was new and interesting in medicine, Donna sought to learn. She has attended medical lectures well into her eighth decade, and constantly refers friends to articles and issues in medicine.

If animals needed surgery, Donna was there to do all the post-operative care and offer the great comfort of her skill to the pet owner. Her retirement gift from her friends had been the sponsorship of a service dog for a wheelchair bound woman. The Canine Companions for Independence program trains the dogs that help those with physical challenges to gain independence, dignity and respect, and so symbolized well all that Donna practiced daily. Once when their own dog needed an intravenous line, Cathy and Donna went to various Emergency Rooms, until Donna had the correct needle and was able to install the line. Donna and Cathy took turns sleeping on the floor with the dog to be sure the animal rested and healed.

Yet, Donna wanted to explore new worlds. Like Milo, she brought to medicine a variety and diversity of talents and skills which she constantly applied on behalf of her patients. Taking a new step in exploration is consistent with her curiosity and the diligence which makes her a consummate healer. What she found and what she has accomplished takes this story both beyond medicine and yet back to the Hippocratic Oath:

With purity and holiness I will pass my life and practice my art.

Chapter VIII

An Anatomist Becomes a Sculptor

In 1988, the Los Angeles Times quoted Donna about the San Diego art scene, beginning with the sign on the reception desk in her office:

> *Part of health is exploring avenues of creative expression.*

Donna told the newspaper:

> *I think that individuals all have various parts of them that need expression. I don't think we should look at people so narrowly in terms of their health, in terms of problems and diseases, which is what specialized medicine is all about. I think it's important to see people as whole, and to support them in the areas of creativity that make them the individuals that they are.*

Los Angeles Times, J Friday, July 1, 1988/Part VI, p 21b

"To see people as whole" could be the summary of Donna's practice of medicine, but now that vision was transferred to her own development as an artist. Mesa Community College offered courses in figurative sculpture. Donna enrolled and quickly exhibited an extraordinary gift. The physician who was teased by her patients for her eager teaching of anatomy, with the help of Dolly, the skeleton, whom she kept in a closet and brought out whenever the opportunity presented itself, now was able to focus on the beauty of the body.

She retired in September of 1991; by July of 1992 she had completed her first 'anatomically correct' figurative sculpture "David Michael" and wrote the description of the Lost

Wax Method of casting in a splendidly illustrated book. A short three years later this sculpture was installed as part of the Boots Cooper, M.D. Memorial Sculpture Garden at the East Falls Campus of Hahnemann University, the heir to Women's Medical College of Pennsylvania. At the dedication, Donna's figure of a little boy is described:

> *"This sculpture of a child is intended to remind us of the life cycle, and of the fact that today's children will be tomorrow's healers."*

We saw in Milo's life that his craftsmanship made playground equipment for children and contributed to his work in prosthetics, as well as his willingness to adapt and restore anything anyone would let him! Donna's sculpture transcended the craft she studied because she is first and foremost a healer, who sees with compassionate vision. Her portrait busts of various friends are alive with affection; we see in the clay the heart of the person represented. Each piece tells a human story; whether she is working on the figure of a young girl, a reclining nude, her own life size self-portrait, or figures of her cat or her dog, the pieces reflect a vision shaped by kindness and caring. The pictures taken of Donna at work reveal not only her intensity of attention, but the surgeon's hands wielding the tools to get just the right fold in an ear, or to create in clay and then bronze the sense of the softness of her cat's fur.

Eleanor Roosevelt wrote:

> *I could not, at any age, be content to take my place by the fireside and simply look on. Life was meant to be lived and curiosity must be kept alive. One must never, for whatever reason, turn his back on life.*

Donna's curiosity has kept her striving for excellence and certainly has driven her achievement as an artist. She has spoken of how the diversity of skills and the variety of engagement necessary to obstetrics is what drew her to that specialization rather than any other, just as Milo wrote of his view that to be a good physician would require that he had the widest possible experience of how people worked and lived. Donna's sculptures are an extension of her curiosity, and an extension of the empathy which is the foundation of her healing.

A surgeon is in some sense a repairman and as such is not only in service to the whole, and to others, but must also begin each task anew, noticing exactly what is amiss, what is unique, and how her skills can fix just what needs fixing without harming the whole. Donna as artist also had to begin each task anew, even as her skills changed and evolved. The skills of a sculptor are deeply related to the skills of a scientist—each requires meticulous observation, each is both technical and deliberative, each can only achieve its ends by a humble reverence to 'knowing' the material world.

When she retired, Donna was given a number of 'awards' by her colleagues, one of which was 'The Most Symmetrical Incision Award'. Donna explains:

> *When the drapes are on the patient, the surgeon cannot see anything in perspective, just the small area that is sterile. So I used to mark everything beforehand, orienting to the hip bones, and making sure I knew the accurate geography.*

This is the surgeon, artist and scientist, as well as the imaginative and empathetic woman speaking. For both Milo and Donna, making is a way of learning. First-hand, personal knowledge enables the maker to transform that knowledge each time something new is made, for something new is learned. Watching Donna create the beauty in which she lives her life, whether by flower arrangements, gardening, or in her joy with friends, the observer sees her making meaning and learning through an ongoing exploration. Her sculpture studio itself is an expression of the form serving the function in a way that expands the vision for those working there, and transforms the dynamic process of work into an adventure. It is a splendid space, perfectly situated overlooking her garden.

For both the sculptor and the scientist, the first step is to know the subject. This is where Donna the anatomist has a great advantage: she sees the bone and sinew beneath the skin, she knows how things can and cannot move; she understands how the layers of flesh grow and decline. However, there are no shortcuts to the intense study of the subject itself. The scientist/artist examines, and reexamines, reflects upon the observations, compares and contrasts perspectives on the subject, and finally recognizes how best to portray the subject. Donna took many photographs of each subject and measured all the landmarks on the body carefully, for her approach to the work is meticulously scientific.

Once the sculptor as scientist had chosen the image, or the representation of the subject, then she must choose the medium. Donna does not work in stone or wood, preferring the accuracy of clay, and the look and feel of the bronze. Building the armature of the piece is the work of an anatomist. In each of her large pieces, Donna's love of anatomy is evident. The building—almost the reverse of a gross anatomy dissection—of the structure of the body is done so that the surface conveys her artistic vision and deep knowledge of the individual portrayed.

Here, too, Donna's training in physical therapy was helpful, for she could indicate both mood and health by the hint of a tensed muscle, or some other small detail most would not notice. Whether nature or nurture or both, Donna's ways of learning hearken back to Milo, who when he began his work in prosthetics, first contacted the engineering department and worked with them to better understand the challenges. Her life size self-portrait bronze is particularly revealing in the subtleties by which Donna the artist has represented Donna the person. She stands, leaning on a shovel, looking down at her garden with profound serenity. One knee is bent, one hand rests on her hip, and we are drawn into the gardener's faith, dedication and work on behalf of all growing things. At any moment we expect the bronze head to look up at us, the eyes to twinkle, and the statue to comment wryly on something we have not yet noticed. As a piece of art, this is exceptional, as a representation of self-knowledge, the portrait is wise and kind and commanding of attention.

Another of her bronzes is 'Ariel" the portrait of a young girl. The making of this piece involved far more than Donna's sculptural talents, for the child's mother was seeking a new path for her life. As she focused on Donna's story she became inspired, understanding at last that being an older student might be an advantage, and that her maturity might make her a better doctor. She is now a renowned Pediatric Radiologist and Oncologist, saying that this is the work she was born to do. The portrait of Ariel conveys not only all the beauty of potential in the child's figure, but an excitement about the life ahead, and what that adventure might be. It has captured a moment of stillness, but we recognize that the girl is about to move onward and upward into her life.

On the web page of Drexel University Medical School, the current affiliate to Women's Medical College of Pennsylvania, there is a discussion of professional formation which states

> *Becoming a physician requires more than the academic mastery of information and technical skills. As physicians, we have to develop our selves. We need to become the kind of person who is a real doctor and healer, capable of acting compassionately, of placing the welfare of our patients above all other considerations, and of caring for those who are medically and socially vulnerable. We need to be the kind of person who can wrestle honestly with all*

> *the psychological, social and financial pressures of medical education and practice and continue to stay close to core values.*
>
> http://webcampus.drexelmed.edu/professionalism/

Donna's art portrays that kind of person, that kind of vision and character.

Donna constantly seeks to learn more about whatever she does. Reflecting now on her years of sculpting she says it is impossible to predict the time necessary to complete a piece, sometimes she could work for four or five hours continuously getting some aspect just right. In surgery as well, there was no real possibility of predicting what might be found and what would be necessary, but Donna would be sure that there was nothing left to accomplish for the patient before she deemed her task finished. Often patients would find her beside them in the recovery room after surgery, as she saw her duty to heal extending far beyond the theater of an operation. Similarly, with the sculpture, each piece is an exegesis, not only an expression of consummate craft. Visitors often reach out to pet the sculpture of Donna's black poodle, even as the lively dog walks by them.

The artist is said to put the hand in service to the eye, so does the surgeon, and behind both the hand and the eye is the heart and mind which seeks to make, or seeks to repair, and by so doing, creates meaning. Donna's office reminded visitors that it was the person who was cared for, and encouraged. Similarly, in her art, Donna conveyed her subject as whole. Milo was known for helping parents of a limb deficient child see that baby as loveable and as a person, not only a deficit. He too created meaning.

Both Milo and Donna came to medicine with a sense of wonder, Donna speaks of the mystery and of the sacred trust the patient gives to the physician. We see that wonder also expressed in Donna's sculpture, for with the finesse of the truly great artists (and surgeons) she is able to portray the beauty and the mystery of living things which fascinate her. Milo had described his own pride in the craftsmanship that went into the building of the Round Barn, or the house for his parents; and Donna was witness to that constant concern whenever as a child she helped Milo in his workshop. Then, as a physical therapist, she experienced the impact on the person's pain and disability by the consistent attention and learning facilitated by the therapist. Layer upon layer of improvement built up to new function, and relief. In her art, the layers of detail build to the whole, and the engagement of the audience, or viewer, becomes part of that reverence.

Sadly, the combination of rheumatoid arthritis and the impact of the long and necessary steroid use on her bone health meant Donna was finding the work in clay increasingly difficult, as was the physical effort of tackling the larger pieces. Making exquisite pieces of jewelry had long been an additional pleasure and gradually Donna concentrated on the less taxing, but equally meticulous craft. At the end of the 1990s, after a decade of retirement, travel, and considerable achievement as an artist, Donna found herself dealing with another aspect of the health care system to which she has dedicated her life: her spine had collapsed, and she was now a patient required by her illness to trust the skill and the courage of other surgeons.

A great deal has been written about role reversals when physicians become patients, and the research has in general concentrated on the increased empathy physicians feel for their patients once they have recovered from an illness. Much less research has examined the physicians who must give up practicing due to illness, and who then must interact over long term debilitation with the changing health care system. One of the assumptions of much of this writing is that the physician ceases to be a physician when ill, that the roles of physician and patient are mutually exclusive.

The training of observation and attention to detail, the scientific drive to examine and explore, and the medical judgment of a physician do not evaporate. Donna remains the trained healer; she is a reflective collaborator in the choices made about her care. It would be false indeed to think that she ignores her training and her commitment to excellence because she does not and cannot treat herself. Her empathy now, however, is directed toward the physicians and nurses who attempt to alleviate her pain and manage the debilitation she has endured.

> *Medicine now follows its reimbursement; physicians are limited by how insurances pay for their time.*

Milo was able to decide to help those who sought his care, no matter what their ability to pay, and Donna established gynecological care for women with disabilities, and worked in free clinics without any payment. Donna's active role as a patient advocate is not a reimbursed role, even though it has drawn on her multiple talents and skills on behalf of hundreds of patients. The changes in the cost of practicing medicine, let alone in attending medical school, have altered the profession Donna loves. She is wistful for the days when medicine was not constrained by legal and insurance issues but was based upon the trust between patient and physician.

Donna feels she was very fortunate: To have practiced both as a solo practitioner, and in partnership when colleagues took the time to build respectful and trusting relationships so that they could discuss their patients in search of quality. Donna was able to maintain her standard of care and standard of caring without determination by an external reimbursement authority. She cannot imagine passing off her patients to the hospital staff and not maintaining her own engagement and responsibility for the patient's care. She remembers the freedom to say 'no' to a patient who asked for an intervention that Donna did not believe was in her best interest, and knows that in practices today the physician's judgment is not paramount in such decisions.

> *A lot changed when insurance companies decided that they would settle claims without consulting the physician. Any such settlement really feels like an admission of culpability, but the choice is just for the company's finances. The physician must be concerned with the best outcome for the patient, not with fear.*

Over the last decade Donna has suffered, as have most patients with chronic complex conditions, from the fragmentation of medicine. Even though her disease affects her whole person, each aspect of that disease is treated by a different specialist. Moreover, rarely do these specialists share their knowledge or their understanding with each other. One may be expert in the impact on her heart of the rheumatoid arthritis, another on the deterioration of bone, another on pain. Donna, the person, who endures, who struggles with the side effects of the medications, and who attempts to coordinate multiple interventions, is not able to gather these physicians and help them understand the whole of her care, let alone the whole of who she is.

> *I think students still enter the profession, or are drawn to it, for the right reasons. I think they need more opportunities, a structure, to share and build a sense of community with each other. Medicine cannot be practiced as a competition with colleagues, or in silence, it must be based on trust for each other as well as trust between the patient and the physician. I feel students are challenged, and discouraged, by the reimbursement systems and constraints they encounter before they have had a chance to build positive relationships.*

With enormous concern for those less able to understand this disease-care system, Donna wonders where the solution lies, and how to help others cope with the challenges.

> *Hospice is a good model of care for the person, but we do not use the model widely enough. There are too many conflicts of interest now, and too little leisure or time to really learn from each other. I am hopeful that we can change things, and optimistic that there will always be some really good physicians dedicated to the art, and to their patients.*

Donna and Cathy have built together a home which is a sanctuary, a haven for healing based not only on the complementarities of the skills of physician and psychotherapist, but on the generosity and respect with which they live their lives. All who come, as guests or as patients, discover in this place of beauty both healing and hope. Strangers want to be immediately adopted into the family, and workmen bring to the home the best of themselves, along with their stories of endurance and struggle. Their lives are lived with constant hospitality and generosity, and their support of many different women in need, extend and expand Donna's practice standards far beyond herself.

Back in 1998, Donna, her student Barbara Levy, and Cathy, a psychotherapist, discussed the question: what was the one thing they would do to change women's health? They agreed that if they could change the impact of starvation imagery which so pervades the media that would have long-term positive effects on women and their choices. Donna and Barb together researched the many clinical impacts and conditions that can be the consequences of a distorted body-image and the attempts to maintain an abstract weight goal. Donna recalled her quiet dismay as a freshman at Pomona when she was measured, and those measurements were taken as an indicator of her value or attractiveness.

From that conversation was born the Real Women Project, a multi-media program which during its decade of operation reached millions of women and spread the message that every woman is more than her body image. Based upon thirteen sculptures of women of all shapes and ages, the project evoked realizations of beauty, of capacity, and of the courage and faith with which women create our world. Formed out of the generosity and skills of the three professionals, the project unified the arts and healing, and opened the minds of all who were exposed to it. Donna had created in her office a place of peace and beauty in which women could find compassionate care and explore their health and capacities. Propelled by Cathy's work and energy, the Real Women Project reached far beyond the location of one medical practice to influence others to establish this public health model of women's health. Donna put her resources and wisdom in service of this effort.

Shortly after one of the first events publicizing the Real Women Project, Donna went in for surgery to fuse her spine. In a photograph taken a few weeks after the surgery, Donna stands with her walker, her body encased in a supporting shell, but she is laughing at the camera, and we see her determination and her excitement about her own healing. In her expression we can see Milo, the maker of prosthetics, Eva the compliant and courageous helper, and Donna, their heir, struggling as she told her patients to 'stand up straight' while she finds something positive to do.

The next project which extended generosity to a national level brought the circle of the tradition back again. Milo had started the work on behalf of limb deficient children, now Donna and Cathy used the stories of Henry, a three-legged cat, to help others learn that it is not the injury or deficiency which defines you, rather it is your response to the experience. This kitten was rescued after the massive forest fires of 2003, and has become a vehicle for outreach conveying the messages that nothing is more disabling than negative attitudes. Again, Cathy's dedication, work and energy gave wings to the idea and it has so far reached several thousand returning veterans and their families, thousands of school children who learn emotional literacy and resilience through animals and over 60,000 exchanges with people who feel safe talking to the cat in ways they would not speak to or through a person. The project materials have been supplied free of cost to the children of Katrina, to many children after the Haiti earthquake, and to military families. The program can be found in Henry's World (www.henrysworld.org), a place that invites healing and evokes recovery from children of all ages, and those who love them. Once again, the public health model of prevention and education unites the arts with healing.

These two national projects represent a consuming effort over the last fifteen years that has engaged extensive resources, time and constant outreach. There is no way to know how many lives have been changed as a result of these projects. The impact extends from a small boy whose leg was amputated, but who gained courage from the story of Henry, to several generations of women who have shared their stories of grief and fear over their own bodies together and have begun for the first time to take steps toward healing. The projects have been produced for the sake of the difference they make, not for any gain experienced by Donna and Cathy. In the truest sense of philanthropy—love of people—these two projects are gifts they have given openly. Similarly they have modeled healing for many aspiring healers and offered intangible and tangible support to students and seekers across the nation.

On a daily basis, it is impossible to predict who will visit, who will call, or what message from a stranger will result in a new step on the journey. Donna supports all the efforts with grace and clarity. When Cathy had to have several surgeries as a result of answering all those letters, Donna the surgeon, Donna the physical therapist, and Donna the loving healer supported and comforted her in every way possible. Cathy is known to be a 'hard stick', meaning her veins roll or disappear making the insertion of a needle difficult for most physicians. More than once, a chagrined anesthesiologist has given up the struggle after many attempts and has gone out to get Dr. Brooks from the waiting room. Donna inserts the needle with no fuss, always successful on the first try.

Despite her physical limitations today, which range from compromised mobility to repeated incidents of heart arrhythmias, Donna reads constantly and maintains her interest in all things medical. She says it is not fair that she has a disease that she did not know about when she was in medical school, referring to rheumatoid lung disease. She voluntarily gave up her medical license because she says she no longer has the keen senses required to be of service. As her medications and illnesses cause her to lose some clarity in executive function, her awareness and empathy keep her deeply connected to others. Her artistry still shows in the flower arrangements which grace her home, and in the way she wraps and decorates the gifts to those she loves. No one and nothing escapes her alert attention: She can see down into the garden from the balcony above and comment on what is blooming and what needs some attention as if she had been on her hands and knees working.

As she looks forward how does she reflect on her legacy?

Chapter IX
What is a Legacy?

In the homesteading world of Milo's youth, no one could know what kind of skills or knowledge would be necessary in dealing with the next challenge. Milo worked the widest possible variety of jobs and each time added skills for future use. He strove to learn and in so doing followed the pioneer tradition, as he created new ways to contribute to others and to the long-term flourishing of his chosen community. In many ways Milo's legacy lies in this constant striving for excellence in order to create something positive in service to others.

Would Milo view his legacy in this same way? In his memoirs of 1981 he wrote that he viewed the Child Amputee Project at UCLA as his legacy; particularly that no child who had need of the services was ever turned away due to lack of ability to pay for the work. At another point, he refers to his work with his students and all the pediatricians from various parts of the world, as equivalent to missionary work which so attracted him in his youth. Throughout the various family reunions, right up until the extensive gatherings of 1983, Milo and Eva rejoiced in the continuity of the family as a legacy of shared values and shared effort.

With older brother Maurice, Milo often praised the tools, the craftsmanship and the disciplines of hard work they had learned, and acquired as a Brooks Family legacy on the farm. They spoke often of their father's admonition that a man could do anything with the right tools. Their parents referred to this tradition and to the imperative of living with 'common sense' as they celebrated various anniversaries up to their seventy-second year of marriage together. In many different obituaries of the family members, two aspects of their lives are consistently highlighted: their loyal duty to the responsibilities within their community, and their faithfulness, expressed either through a church or through their own dedication to service.

Rena Brooks, especially, praised the family legacy of striving for education and of using that education in service to others. More than the other siblings, Rena's writings have a real sense of sharing a perspective on behalf of the heirs of the family traditions. In 1974, when both Rena and Frances died, the obituaries point out that Rena, who was born in 1892, graduated from teachers' college, so was a pioneer of women's education for her time. It was Rena who commented on the skills and common practicality necessary to the moon landing as she watched it.

The Brooks family exhibits the quintessential virtues of the homesteaders of the West: With faith and fortitude and mutual aid they overcame or adapted to the external threats while working toward the imagined world that would survive and thrive at some time in the future. The family members each took responsibility for learning what was necessary to contribute to their communities, and they dealt with each other with transparent integrity. The Brooks children and grandchildren trusted each other to do as they said they would do, and the community bore witness to that trust not only in the various reunions, but in the *Brooks Babbler*'s remarkable continuity of real communication.

Perhaps the most adventuresome of Melvina's grandchildren was Robert Tracy, Delia's son, who became the founder of Tracy Seeds, producing seeds for agricultural production, which at one point was the largest seed company in South America, as well as in the Midwest. In 2013, Robert's grandson Josh has revived Tracy Seeds, keeping the century-old farming tradition alive. Bob Tracy was a frequent and lengthy contributor to the *Brooks Babbler*, and his various aunts and uncles and cousins were intrigued by his international work and travel, just as they were intrigued by Milo, whom some called 'the famous brother' with typical sibling teasing. Robert Tracy's letters to the *Babbler* about his travels in Africa and South America especially as the tries to help other farmers are filled with reflection on the traditions of the Midwest. He constantly says "we should be so grateful for what we have and what we know" and his gratitude is certainly reflected in the generosity of his work.

Striking to any reader outside the family is how much detail of their lives the writers share in the *Brooks Babbler.* Not only do the contributors write with confidence that others are interested in the details of their lives, but they write in an expectation of shared learning. Milo is often sent medical details of relatives he will not see as a physician while others share architectural drawings or comments on raising livestock. The family forum is a continuous learning enterprise; when one member speaks of retirement communities and real estate prices in Florida, another will compare those issues with what is available in Arizona, or Palm Springs, California. The news is shared as if they were gathered around a picnic blanket or sitting in a school room waiting to discuss some matter critical to their town. The discussions are among siblings and grandchildren, but the tone is that of committed citizens, responsible for shaping a future.

As was evident in the stories of Milo Brooks' life, he was a deeply reflective man; each of the major life events cause him to wonder aloud about the purpose and lesson he must draw. The legacy of a pioneering family creates continuous meaning for the heirs, in a variety of ways. Milo found meaning in service to his calling, as a physician, as a creator of new solutions, and as a servant of his community. Although he was frequently recognized for his many accomplishments, Milo often expresses gratitude for the life he has lived, for his opportunities, and for the love and support of Eva and of the rest of the family. This sense of good fortune pervades the family, and we must be reminded of the struggles they transcended: from prairie fire, to desperate winters, to poverty and lack of opportunity, to untimely deaths and long illnesses, to the sorrows of wars and the decisions consequent to failures of crops and of businesses.

Accomplishment does not mean recognition; rather it is the 'making something of oneself' which matters to the pioneers. The homesteading tradition was not supportive, or tolerant of anyone who wished to sit on the sidelines. We saw how eager Milo was 'for something positive to do', and each time he set himself a goal—such as making playground equipment for Donna and Ron's school—he gave it his best effort. We sympathize with Eva over the possums in the backyard, but we understand the goal to find out more about the care of premature babies which drove that experiment.

Milo the craftsman, as well as Milo the researcher, was consistently curious to create something new. He speaks of the Child Amputee Project as his 'lasting contribution' and he reflects often on how new and exciting the work is as it attracts physicians and nurses from around the world. As a teenager, Milo felt that same exhilaration with the making of the Round Barn: it was something very new and different, and every aspect required consummate craftsmanship and shared skill. Donna recalls that each time she returned home to visit during her student years, her father wanted her to come to his workshop to see whatever new project he was working on. Work in all aspects was creation, and that meant both fulfillment of duty and connection to others.

Duty is an old fashioned word in 2013, but it was at the core of the Brooks tradition over generations. Maurice recalled the duty of getting his sisters safely home from school in a white out blizzard on the prairie, Milo took great joy at age ten when he could 'do the work of a man' and thus contribute to the family. As physicians, both Milo and Donna put the duty to care for their patients far above any financial gain from their work. Eva and Milo opened their home to many students and international visitors as both a duty and as a gesture of gratitude for their own good fortune.

Rena's praise of the striving for education common among the siblings was echoed in Milo's delight in expanding opportunities for learning. Whether he is visiting other pediatricians in America or seeing what care is like on another continent, Milo repeatedly says "it was a great chance for learning". There are frequent statements in his memoirs such as "I learned a lot," and we feel Milo's drive for clear understanding and for constantly improving practical solutions to whatever he encounters. When Donna establishes her practice, he wants to rehang the doors on the cupboards so that they function better, as when Thalidomide children are treated, he wants to find better ways to help them live fully. Nothing escapes his notice, or his effort to improve his skills.

Milo's daughter Donna exemplifies the same passion to know more and be better able to understand whatever it is she is dealing with. We are reminded of Melvina again and her guidance "strive to understand", and of the fact that as soon as the opportunity to learn to read (with her eldest child) presented itself, Melvina eagerly took advantage of it.

Part of the legacy of homesteaders, including the Brooks family, is their resilience in the face of tragedy and loss. Ellsworth, the father of the family, endured crop failures and business failures, and eventually had to leave the family homestead in order to support the family as someone's employee. Milo had to work at jobs that put his life in constant danger in order to go to school, and even then, he had to take long breaks from study in order to save money to pay the tuition. Yet, even after the untimely death of children, or the unexpected destruction of a dream, we do not hear from Milo and his family any bitterness or complaint. They may as they age express frustration with some of their losses of function—Julia complains when her children want her to stop driving, and Milo regrets that he does not have the stamina at eighty-three that he had even ten years before—but these are frustrations, not anger. Donna certainly regrets her physical losses, but with a wistful serenity, not bitterness.

In studies of what contributes to the building of resilience or adaptive strength, we know that both the stimulation for learning and the inspiring and protective roles of models and mentors are keys to a child's sense of mastery and confidence. Despite the physical hardships of the homestead, we know that it was a richly stimulating environment, and that adults were both conscious and responsible in their roles as mentors. These children lived as apprentices not only of how to survive, but of how to live in a skillful manner, and Milo wrote eloquently of his gratitude to his father for teaching him to be a craftsman. When Milo decided that the time had come to do something in return for his parents, as many of the siblings as possible helped with the building of the Hardin house. Milo wrote with great admiration and gratitude of the several mentors he found in medicine, just as Donna found women mentors both at Rancho los Amigos, and at the Women's Medical College of Pennsylvania.

Both Milo and Donna became mentors and role models to others, and took that responsibility seriously, again sacrificing personal gain in order to help a new physician become successful, or a patient to thrive. Yet it is interesting that Milo and Donna denied that he was a role model to her. Certainly, Milo would not have wished anyone to think that Donna had entered medicine by riding on his coattails: Not only did he have more respect for her than that would imply, but he had a profound belief that each person should be trusted and supported to pursue their own choices and destiny. This was very much a homesteader's view: People could only bootstrap themselves, once their choice was made however, everyone could help as needed.

Donna has been acutely aware of her role as a mentor to young women physicians, given the timing of her own entry when women were a mere 7% of the profession, and given the need to model the pursuit of excellence and empathy to which she was and is so profoundly committed. Just as Milo used his positions in academic medicine to introduce students and colleagues to the art of treating limb deficient children, Donna used her clinical practice and referrals to help others in practice and to model the kind of practice where women feel secure and encouraged to understand their own health. Donna has been the epitome of generous care and support given to any who need it, and thus is the heir of the pioneer women across the west who established communities based on generosity.

In contrast, our contemporary society often seems to speak of what is 'deserved', whether that is in advertising slogans or political acrimony. For Milo and Donna, what has always mattered is 'need', whether that is a clinical need or a human need. Milo first started accepting multiple jobs at his various educational institutions because they had a need and could find no one willing to work hard enough to address it. On a farm, just as in a solo medical practice, you address the task in front of you and complete it so that then you can move to the next task. As Donna says of surgery, you look to solve what is immediate, and you do not leave the site until you have done all that you can do. Repeatedly, in Milo's and Maurice's memoirs, we see that it was the task at hand which governed the work of the farm, long-term plans depended on too many uncontrollable factors to overrule immediate need.

This is not to say that there were no long-term plans: Milo worked to escape the farm life and then to become the best pediatrician and educator he could become through decades of struggle. Donna worked to be able to be the best and most effective physician to the needs of women that she could, moving from her physical therapy career on to her expertise as a surgeon. Even the earliest records of the Brooks ancestors cite the family motto as "By Persevering".

One of the aspects of resilience which appears to be a personality characteristic rather than a skill is practical intelligence: an ability to apply what one knows to living, to daily life. Milo the carpenter built barns and houses and playground equipment and prosthetics; he praised both his tools and his teachers right until the last years of his life. His delight in the retirement community was significantly influenced by the fact that he found there a workshop better than in his own home. While he may have travelled to Heidelberg and Japan to examine ways of dealing with limb deficiencies, he was never inhibited by his own status and reputation from taking out his tools and putting them to work. Eva's letters often tell us that Milo 'can hardly wait' to start fixing things for others.

Donna the anatomist became a proficient physical therapist helping polio patients learn to function again, became a surgeon, then when she had to withdraw from that practice, became an accomplished sculptor, expanding her view of medicine to a broad and inclusive public health approach. Her skills kept developing, and whenever external factors complicated her life, she applied them in order to transcend and transform her life and the lives of others.

The Brooks siblings and grandchildren seem to have this practical intelligence in abundance. Yet they reinforced each other's talents with constant communication and encouragement through seven decades of the *Babbler.* Imagine the sense of belonging felt by the young couple setting forth from rural Wisconsin on their honeymoon trip, knowing that they could come out to the Pacific coast and return, welcomed at every stop by a member of the family. The *Babbler* recounts repeatedly the delight in many young couples visits that the older family experienced , and we see the sense of passing on both tradition and deep love as treasured heirlooms are given to this new couple. Sometimes the Brooks family seems a bit like an Old Testament record of an intensely interesting tribe, and Milo occasionally is like the son sent away from the farm to succeed and bring back his knowledge. Equally often he is teased for his desire to be involved in everything:

when Rena and her family are settling in to retirement in Arizona, Rena writes that Milo has asked that some of the renovation and building be 'saved' for him to do.

It is the knowledge shared which indicates success to this family, and especially knowledge applied in service to others. Often we think legacy means merely a tangible gift, but for most of our ancestors, legacy was intangible: the lessons from lives lived on behalf of the future. Donna has been consistently generous with her tangible assets, supporting scholarships, projects and her various professional associations, but this can hardly be construed as the most important aspect of her legacy.

Barbara Levy M.D. is Vice-President for Health Policy at the American College of Obstetricians and Gynecologists. In her first year of medical school she was assigned to Dr. Donna Brooks, ostensibly for a rotation lasting a quarter of a year. Donna became Barb's mentor and guide.

> *She embraced me and we recognized in each other our dedication to patients. Donna saw a seed in me and nourished it and fed it and guided my growth. Donna lived and breathed a total commitment to patients and to the practice of medicine. Everything from her demeanor to her interactions with patients to her relationships with other physicians expressed her dedication.*

At the time, Barb was thinking of entering family practice, but that soon changed.

> *Donna gently suggested that women needed other women in order to gain really good care, and she made a compelling argument that if I entered obstetrics and gynecology I could become a comprehensive physician, doing all the things required in primary care but being a surgeon and an obstetrician as well.*

What was to have been just a rotation has become a lifelong treasured friendship based upon mutual respect and shared passion. Donna would alert Barb to an interesting case, and if it were possible the student would join the surgeon for yet another opportunity to learn.

> *I felt welcomed in her practice at any time, she made it possible for me to be absorbed by the practice of women's health care. Donna was able to see what my professional growth needed and guided me to that.*

The relationship did not really change after Barb Levy graduated, but deepened and expanded as their lives changed. Now, having achieved a position of influence, Barb still feels her apprenticeship to Donna was fundamental to the kind of doctor she has become. Today she feels that it is Donna's love of life and of people which makes her so exceptional.

> *Donna naturally worked as part of a team with the nurses and the other physicians each contributing their best in their specific roles. This is what works out to be the best advantage for our patients. Donna always reinforced the respect and the love which is true caring.*

Barb Levy agrees with Donna that she was fortunate to retire when she did because of the autonomy possible then for a primary care physician, and because it was still possible financially to sustain that kind of practice. When she thinks of Donna's legacy, Barb says:

> *The legacy began with Donna's father and the grounded professionalism and dedication to service that she learned. She then taught me to love the art and the science of medicine, she modeled and taught it and now my daughter embraces those standards and that dedication as she practices as a physician.*

Chapter X

The Traditions of Care

When Milo Brooks began his long quest to become a physician, he faced years of hardship, diverse and challenging work, and the constant discipline of saving in order to achieve his goal and his purpose. When he observed mistakes made in taking a history in the Emergency Room, he recognized that a true physician must understand the context of patient's lives and the vocabulary that was meaningful to each patient. He knew that he would have to apply his medical knowledge to many individuals who could not describe why they needed his help in specific clinical terms. His quest thus became an expansive gathering of specific knowledge and adaptive skills. His history shows us the continuity of the practical knowledge of the homestead: Nothing learned was ever wasted.

Donna's training to be a healer began when, as a child, she accompanied her father on rounds, or sterilized his instruments, or sharpened the needles. Her natural curiosity drove her to understand what she was doing and how to do it better. She reflects now on the ways she has been treated as a patient by an array of specialists.

> *You have to use common sense about interventions. It is important not to do something immediately but to wait and watch and learn. You have to trust the tincture of time, and know when an intervention will be truly helpful.*

When she first encountered a patient, Donna would ask "How may I be helpful to you?", as Milo when first meeting the parents of a limb deficient child would say "What a beautiful baby you have!" Neither began with anything other than an attitude of service, and both Milo and Donna began to build a relationship with each patient based on empathy. One of the specialists who now treats Donna worries deeply about the young residents she teaches. She feels there has been a change in their expectations so that the students she sees do not seem dedicated to following their patients, or preparing ahead of a visit , but rather expect the authority and respect to come with the role, not due to their own behavior in relationship with others.

She is concerned that this leads to assumptions of a doctor's 'rights' rather than to the responsibilities of real service.

Milo and Donna were 'mature' students in today's language, both had worked and learned and been responsible and accountable adults before they entered medical school. Donna feels strongly that her practice as a physical therapist gave her a great advantage once she reached medical school, not only because she knew a lot about anatomy and the principles of movement, but because she knew how to build a relationship with a patient. In physical therapy, both the patient and the therapist can see and experience the impact of care, and can watch and learn how the body is healing through how movement is possible. Donna also believes that her years in physical therapy reinforced her commitment to preventive care.

> *Many long term problems are preventable, such as decubiti, (bed sores) there is no excuse for them, they are entirely preventable, but people think they are inevitable.*

Pregnancy may be the most important window for learning for both a mother and her unborn baby, as the woman is usually ready, eager and attentive to what the doctor has to teach. Donna laments the current constraints on a physician in which insurance companies measure a physician's productivity in terms of patient 'encounters' and thus may pressure the doctor to spend less than seven minutes with each patient. (The range in the US is from 6 to 18 minutes per patient.) This diminishes the physician's role as an educator and compromises the building of a relationship which Donna and Milo felt was critical to good care. It also allows no time for discussions of preventive behaviors or the context of illness or distress.

How can our lessons learned from Donna and Milo identify some of the needed changes in medical education and in medical practice?

Currently students are accepted into medical school based on their test scores and personal essays, with final decisions based on the interview with an admissions committee. However, those who sit on the committee are not necessarily in clinical practice and may have not been accountable for patient care outside of the hospital. For a long time schools have apparently searched for those who will 'perform' well, especially under the pressures of workload and competition, rather than those who seek to serve, and who combine kindness with humility. Donna and Milo not only shared the fact that they were mature individuals of proven character before they entered medical school, but they had also known and endured some of the pains of the human condition: both in families that knew loss, and by being alert to the struggles of those around them.

Both were exceptionally disciplined students, maintaining their academic excellence against the odds of circumstances. Both had already learned time management by having to work and study at the same time; neither had lived free of financial worries. Milo in fact worked to pay for his studies in cash; Donna maintained her standing in order to retain her scholarships. How the extreme debt load incurred by most current medical students impacts the ways they practice medicine after graduation has not been extensively studied. We do know that it is the financially rewarded specialties rather than primary care which attract most medical students. Both Milo and Donna were attracted to pediatrics and obstetrics/gynecology respectively because of the variety of challenges and skills required of the physician in primary care.

In Milo's time and for Donna at Women's Medical College of Pennsylvania, the model of teaching was the apprenticeship model. Students were mentored as human beings in their journey to become doctors, and they were able to watch and model themselves after their teachers with whom they established a personal relationship. With the standardization of examinations and licensure requirements, less emphasis has been placed in recent decades on this apprenticeship engagement in mutual learning. Further, mentorship is often treated as a recruitment tool with high school outreach to increase the diversity of a student body. Thus it is not often cultivated as an engagement outside the teaching institution, or by the practicing clinician.

Milo and Donna went on a variety of rounds, on home visits, and to community health locations as part of their education. The short duration of clinical rotations which usually begin in the third year of medical school, rarely offers the student or the physician the opportunity to build a lasting relationship through which both can learn. If the mentoring doctor is to inspire the student, they must face diverse challenges together and the student must be ready to learn, not merely by fulfilling one more requirement in a long and wearing test of endurance.

A decade ago there was a movement to have medical students admitted as patients and subjected to the same routines as someone with a specific diagnosis admitted to the hospital. The Learning by Living project has students who are interested in a specialty in geriatrics spend two weeks as a patient in a nursing home. However, these efforts have been voluntary and have not been widely integrated into a standard curriculum. Current research has established that medical student's empathy declines during the time spent in medical school and takes its most significant drop in the third year just as students begin patient care.

Donna comments:

> *Students enter medical school often with high ideals, and many truly want to help others, but schooling teaches them to be preoccupied by huge amounts of textbook learning and to fear not knowing something. We should help them engage with a practicing physician from the very first day in medical school. That way they could really get to know what patient care involves, they could learn to prepare and to follow a patient over time, they could learn to listen and to watch and to really observe the little details. The practicing physician would be showing them what the textbook knowledge really means.*

Milo had no tolerance for a medical student who wanted to go to lunch before telling the parents of a sick child how their child was doing, and he raged (on paper in his memoirs) about physicians who did not include the family in their discussions of treatment, follow-up and prevention. He often accompanied a family to the hospital and through the admission process after making a first diagnosis on a home visit. Similarly, Donna as patient advocate has accompanied individuals through diagnosis, treatment and recovery, and still is vigilant to be sure that those dealing with a medical crisis understand what is being said or done. For both Milo and Donna their learning as apprentices naturally evolved into their becoming mentors of younger, aspiring doctors, and both felt this as an obligation to their craft.

Milo often reflected on the ways that skills and tools were passed on across the generations from his homesteading grandparents, and he clearly grasped each opportunity to build, repair and create with young people at the family reunions, the YMCA, and through Rotary student exchanges. Donna is quick to encourage those seeking a medical career, and continues to inspire those who meet her, but she is cautious about how much can be taught in the institutional setting, and how much must be learned by doing.

> *There are different ways to learn, and a few medical schools are offering alternatives to the lecture style. Problem-based learning with a clinical case is a good beginning, but I think it should be with practicing clinicians, not only academic physicians. We have to do a better job teaching collaboration and teamwork.*

Let us reflect a little on the building of the Round Barn in 1914, one of the pivotal experiences of Milo's childhood. Donna says it was referred to often in the family. We do not know why E.E. Brooks, Milo's father, chose to build a round barn. He was a taciturn man, but we know he took enormous pride in craftsmanship. The barn-raising was directed by the architect and those who had built such a barn before, but all of the community helped. The volunteer labor was part of the mutual aid and mutual responsibility of the homestead.

Milo and his siblings all participated to the best of their abilities; if they were too young to contribute more than fetching and carrying materials, they were certainly expected to be watching and learning. Examinations on the homestead were much harder than those in the classroom, for these examinations were the next tasks—the ability to address the next similar problem. Further, the test of the barn-raising was time—how long was the barn useful, and how long did it stand. The Brooks round barn was finally destroyed in 1995 after serving for eighty-one years.

Donna learned, and taught, surgery in a similar way: Those in charge were those who had done the task before, but everyone around had to help to the best of their ability. In Donna's practice, as with a barn-raising, you could not scrub in to participate unless you had done the detailed work of a history and physical examination so that you were fully prepared in your knowledge of the patient.

Yet there is an important caveat: Medical knowledge is changing rapidly—what the student learns from a textbook in first year, may be outdated and replaced by new knowledge by the fourth year of medical school. Thus, it is not the knowledge or data which is critical to creating a good physician: It is the willingness to learn and the skills that apply that ever-changing knowledge. In the barn-raising, the knowledge of how was no more important than the knowledge of where and what for, that too changed as the community changed. In teaching her students, Donna established preparation, attentiveness and skilled practice were fundamental, but they had to be applied with others, and they had to report what they were doing, or had done, or planned to do, with clarity.

Both Milo and Donna were hands-on practitioners, using their clinical skills, as well as the comfort and reassurance of touch. In the old photographs of Milo at the family reunions, we see glimpses of him as he holds an infant relative or squats to talk with a great-niece or nephew. This is the pediatrician meeting the child as a human being with his attitude of care obvious at once. Similarly, the proud pictures of Donna with the infants she delivered show her delight in the family's happiness.

One of the shared themes in the lives of father and daughter is that of gratitude. Both Milo and Donna frequently expressed gratitude for their good fortune at being able to practice medicine as they did. Milo's letter to the *Brooks Babbler* after the fire destroyed his home is quintessential: meaning is found in the human relationships of the present moment, what matters is not what is gone, but what is shared. When Donna speaks of her busy practice now, it is with a profound gratitude for the relationships, and as she says "the privilege of serving".

Milo and Donna maintained an optimistic view and serenity even when faced with heart-wrenching challenges. We know that Milo's sense of failure regarding his son Richard's death shaped his practice of medicine, but there is no evidence that he lost his ability to seek positive action with a positive attitude. Similarly, when Donna's rheumatoid arthritis forced her retirement, she found a new avenue for her skills and sought new ways to apply her knowledge. In some ways she is even grateful that her disease has spared her having to confront the deterioration she perceives in the ways medicine is now practiced.

> *Hospitals and medical schools need to make it possible for clinicians to meet and talks as colleagues, without pressures of reimbursement or time management. Conversations lead to cooperation, and we need more of that.*

Milo participated in these conversations well into his eighties and took delight in the young physicians who were present to learn and contribute. Donna in retirement has attended many medical meetings and gatherings to keep her knowledge current, and to sustain this important conversation. As medicine has come to be analyzed as a 'delivery system' and the metrics of 'throughput' used to assess physician 'performance', real conversation let alone meaningful feedback, has been crowded out of practice. Not only does this have ongoing adverse consequences for patients— as Donna experiences when her several specialists do not communicate with each other— but it has a negative influence on the maturation and wholeness of the physician as a human being.

Milo not only had Eva's stability and support to engage him beyond his clinical commitments, he maintained close ties with several community organizations such as Rotary, the YMCA and his church. He was therefore not isolated. His understanding of people was embedded in his own involvements with diverse groups and diverse responsibilities. From his earliest years after leaving the farm, we saw that Milo taught Sunday School, was engaged in sports and befriended many people in many different livelihoods. With his large group of siblings and the consistency of the *Brooks Babbler*, he was able to maintain ties that constantly required that he explain medical changes to lay people who were not his patients, and to be involved in the broader concerns of his community. Donna has maintained a variety of interests and involvements over the years, leading to her careers as a sculptor and artist, as a patient advocate, and as a philanthropist. Her home is busy with visitors and friends, and she has used computers to keep in touch, and play a wicked game of Scrabble with those who cannot visit. She regularly plays bridge and avidly enjoys musical theater. Neither Milo nor Donna perceived medicine as separate from this wide variety of engagements. Each paid alert attention to the dimensions of living that cannot be counted or measured.

There is in this way of living a dignity which sometimes seems lost to us. We call those who lived through the Depression and WWII "The Greatest Generation" and grieve a cultural loss as they die. Our press and media exaggerate the supposed 'rugged individualism' of America, without grasping the rugged engagement in community of our pioneers, exemplified in the Brooks family traditions. Donna and Milo applied those traditions to medical practice thereby enriching both the practice and the traditions they shared. The fragmentation of our current medical care industry not only diminishes all participants from patients to administrators to nurses and physicians by imposing inappropriate measures and expectations on what must be an intimate trust, but it isolates each of these participants from the nurture and dignity of membership in a mutually beneficial community. Milo and Donna worked hard to maintain their ties to this broad community, ranging from their participation in the regular Brooks family reunions which were really loving explorations of how the members were flourishing, to their own continuous engagement in learning and the diverse human experience.

Wisdom is not scarce in our world, but it is often hard to discover and develop. Often the wise among us live as does Donna, invisible to the world of broad accolades preferring to make her contributions in terms of the dignity and professing of healing in the relationships she cultivates. Milo received many awards for his teaching and work, but what he prized was the love of Eva, and the compassion and kindness he saw in his daughter as Donna practiced their shared calling.

Broad surveys of patients asking what constitutes good care inevitably list kindness first. Similar surveys asking what makes a good physician list kindness first, followed by humility. Donna's humility leads her to recognize the excellence and achievements of her students and patients with pride, but she sees herself as driven to seek excellence rather than as having achieved it. Milo rose to his professorships with constant long hours spent away from his family and with a lifelong appetite for learning. When recognition came to him, he shared it, knowing that his ability to work depended on the contributions of others. Frequently in the *Brooks Babbler* one of the far flung members of the family will thank Milo, or Donna, for their call, or for their note of concern and kindness during a crisis or an illness. The family sometimes reacts with surprise at their own traditions, and praise Milo and Donna for having helped someone in the extended family at the same time that they themselves are reaching out. Just as Eva and Milo were generous with their hospitality to students, family members and professional colleagues from around the globe, so the appreciation from these beneficiaries usually begins with reference to kindness.

Says Barb Levy:

> *I don't believe you can be a good doctor if you do not love people. Donna truly loves people.*

Donna feels the key to being a good physician is empathy. Milo would say it included a loving curiosity. To Barb Levy it is exactly this dedication and sense of service which is being lost as young physicians seek a more 'balanced' life.

> *I think we have gone too far in that direction and we are becoming a trade rather than a profession, as young physicians' own personal interest trumps the dedication to patients and to medicine. Handing off a patient to the care of a hospitalist, or someone else's shift would not have happened in Donna's practice.*

She agrees with Donna, that young students need to have mentors in clinical practice. The real difficulty is to find the physicians willing and able to model dedicated service.

> *Many schools make a real effort in the first two years to teach students a humane approach, that they are treating a person not a body part, but as soon as they are in the hospital, what is modeled is the fragmented specialization and 'mindless' rushing which is not good for the profession, or for our patients. Since physicians are measured by productivity, there is no time to talk, no time to reflect.*
>
> *We live and practice in a time of litigation and we live in a culture that expects us to be all things for all people at all times, so we practice in fear that we may miss the one thing out of five million other things. We forget that we do not have to make every decision this minute, we can revisit our choices, we can adapt our treatment plans, but that requires that we have had time to develop a relationship and a trust with our patients.*

One of Donna's colleagues, JoLeah von Herzen, M.D., emphasizes how important it was to Donna that she educate her patients and spend time explaining, listening and reviewing until she was confident that her patient understood all that was going on. JoLeah says "Empathy is not much use unless you know how to communicate that, and Donna was a great listener, always able to convey her interest and her caring."

> *She's a really good thinker, she can problem solve and think something through with her colleagues so everyone on the team knows what to do. She was always thinking ahead, getting us ready for what might happen or what was the next step. She did not have to help see that the unit in the hospital was running well, but she always helped the nurses manage and plan. She was generous to all of us in helping out.*

This is once again the practical intelligence that was so important on the farm, so important to Milo as well. The broad understanding of what it took to deliver what was best for the patient engaged Donna and Milo far beyond a specific clinical intervention. So too is the teamwork, the mutual aid and generosity, which were hallmarks of the homestead as they became hallmarks of clinical practice for both Milo and Donna. Each person was trained to contribute, and that contribution had to be appreciated, recognized and encouraged. Barb Levy says that Donna was always a very loving employer, and JoLeah says "She could be stern, and demanding, and never did anyone slack off around her, but she made our work fun, she was so willing to help each one of us."

JoLeah remembers Donna talking about Milo's work with limb deficient children:

> *Donna said her Dad told her that a patient listens carefully to every word you say about the newborn baby, and you can shape how the mother will treat the child and view the child by what you say. He felt that you must always speak to give hope, to give confidence, so that the baby is viewed as the important person she will become.*

Since patients were often awake during a C-Section, Donna was very strict about what was said in the operating room; one young doctor taped his mouth shut the second time he scrubbed in with Donna, for the first time he had said "Oops" during the surgery. Donna was not pleased.

JoLeah remembers Donna's standards as demanding, and says

> *She was extremely fair with colleagues, she started paying me for the deliveries I did when she was travelling, saying it was not fair to take for granted the time that was required. I loved working with her, and if she said to me, "Good job, Babe," I felt totally encouraged.*

As part of her obligation to understand and then to educate the patient, Donna would talk to the authors of various reports—the radiologist, or the pathologist—and ask for their opinion on the case. Now, says JoLeah, very few doctors take the time to dig in to the report and really understand what is being said or implied. In addition, Donna insisted on having good photographs of each surgery so that she could show the patient what the reality was, and what she had done.

> *"We always had medical students around," says JoLeah. "Donna was totally committed to teaching them and encouraging them. She made time for them and she made sure they had real opportunities to learn.*
>
> *Women doctors were not very well treated when we began working together, but Donna initiated real respect for the female physicians in the San Diego community. She had very good relationships with the staff wherever she practiced, and she got a lot of referrals because of the respect we all had for her. She has really good clinical judgment. With Donna you were encouraged to be on the team and to do your very best. It is sad that that has changed now.*

The measures of physician performance and productivity today do not take into account the 'good clinical judgment'. Again, the constraints upon the time spent with the patient often mean that the physician cannot take the time to exercise that judgment, but does what is both defensive and fearful. Donna remembers that the first woman OB/ Gyn physician in San Diego, Katherine Carson, had been an outspoken activist for women, fighting the battles loudly and with very clear passion.

> *"I took a different approach. I wanted to practice as an example and achieve my reputation by precepting," Donna remembers.*

It did not take long for her patient load to be filled. Once when a psychotherapist was seeking a new gynecologist, she told an anesthesiologist friend that she had made an initial appointment with Dr. Donna Brooks. He asked her to wait until he checked to find out who was the very best. He said after his research "You already have the best doctor."

Milo knew many of his patients as his neighbors in his own community, Donna treated some of her patients through decades of living, and then treated their children and friends and neighbors. Each person was remembered as unique, and their story known. As Donna now looks at the pictures of her with newborns, she knows what has become of the little girl or boy. She is part of their story and each story continues.

For every doctor, one of the greatest challenges is facing and accepting failure, loss and the inability to make a difference for the patient. Milo carried this grief and a sense of shame with him as a result of Richard's death and said he dealt with it by a sense that he must "just keep going" despite being unable to help Eva and his other children. For Donna, the greatest challenge is her frightening loss of mental clarity and her fluent thinking and memory. She watched her mother vanish as a person through the tragedy of Alzheimer's disease, and she wishes to spare those who love her some of the hard decisions she herself had to make. She comments "If I didn't understand and accept my cognitive limitations I would not be able to live with my inability to no longer do service." Yet it is another lesson in service that she is open and accepting of this reality, and of the consequences of her decline. She exemplifies in this what makes a good doctor a great doctor: she is responsible not to mislead others, not to pretend that she can do things she no longer can do. She voluntarily gave up both her medical license and her driver's license, so that she would 'do no harm'. Further, there is greatness in Donna's wisdom in recognizing that she tires easily and cannot maintain focus, so that she accepts what cannot be changed. Many doctors, sometimes called 'heroic', keep intervening even though they know their efforts are futile and will not help. Donna refuses to betray her calling or herself, and thus remains, above all, an example of what makes a physician a healer.

When Donna was elected to the medical honor society, Alpha Omega Alpha, she learned that the organization's motto was "Be Worthy to Serve the Suffering". The motto succinctly summarizes the moral position of Milo and Donna. To each of them in both similar and different ways, the calling of medicine required that they as human beings exemplified what they practiced as physicians. Donna hears the grief about where medicine is today expressed by so many physicians, and she is nostalgic for the 'golden age' of service. However, being Melvina's granddaughter, and living with her constant alert attention to what is possible, Donna knows as long as there are new models of care, there are new frontiers to be explored.

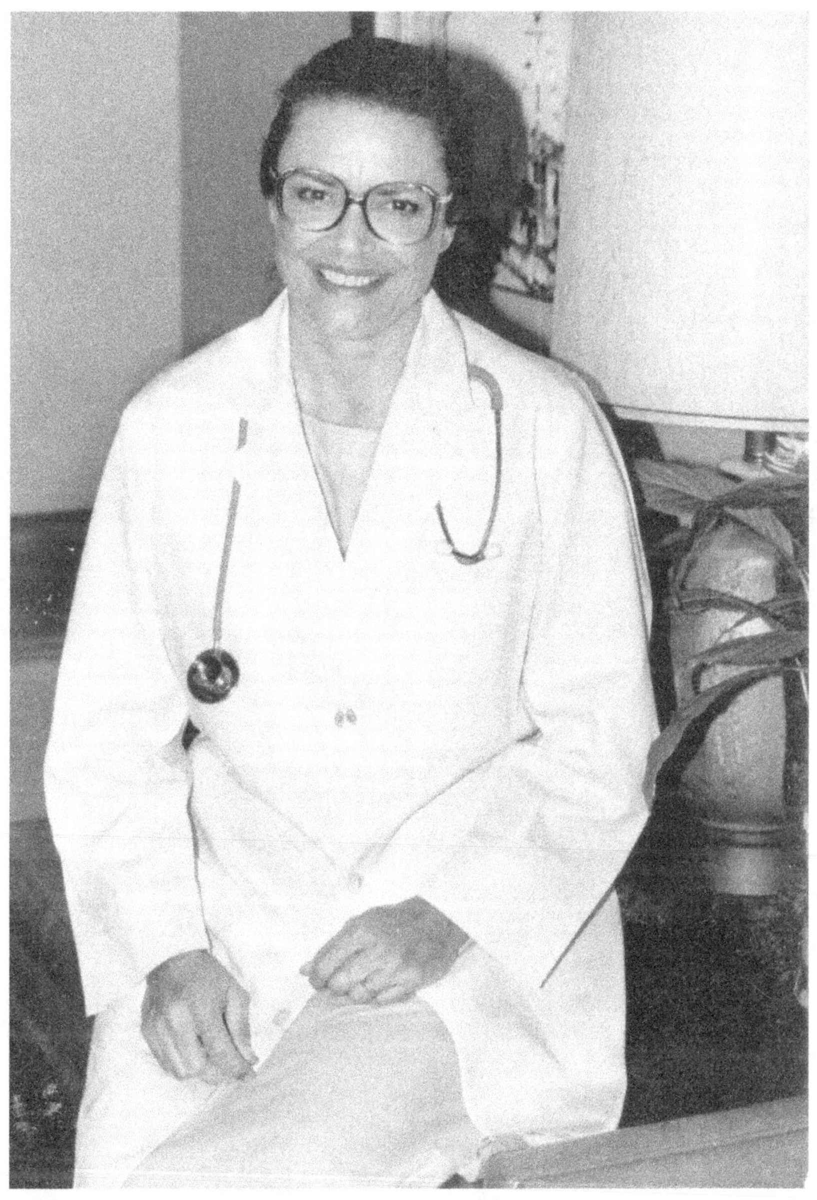

Donna at the office, taken by Nea Fen, a patient

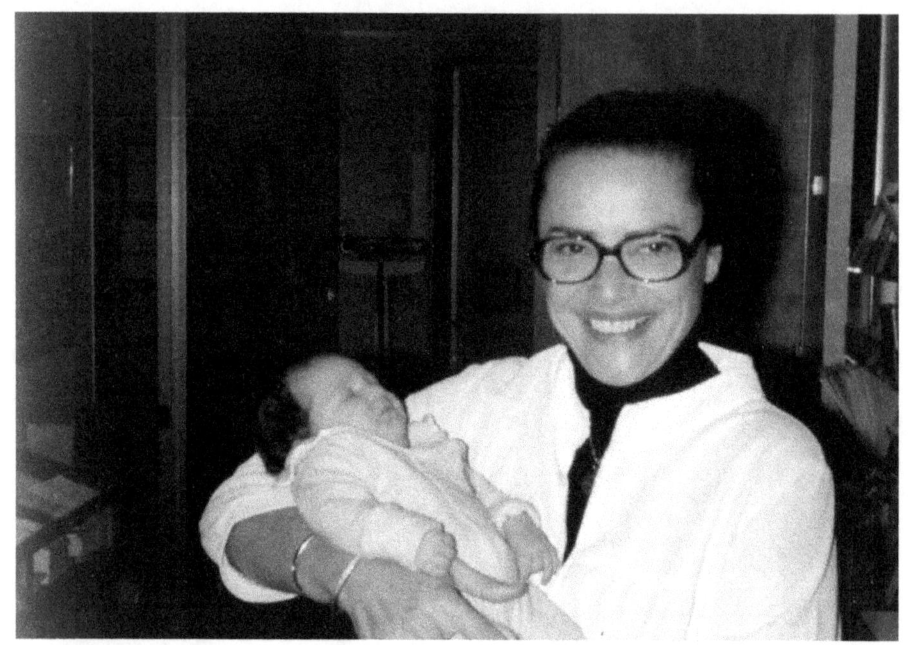

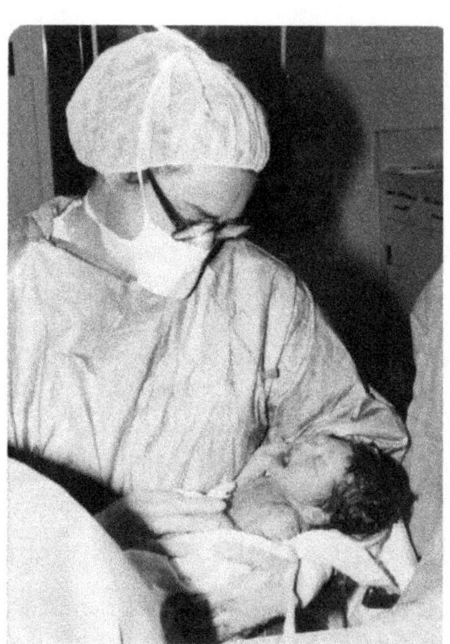

Two newborns and their delighted obstetrician

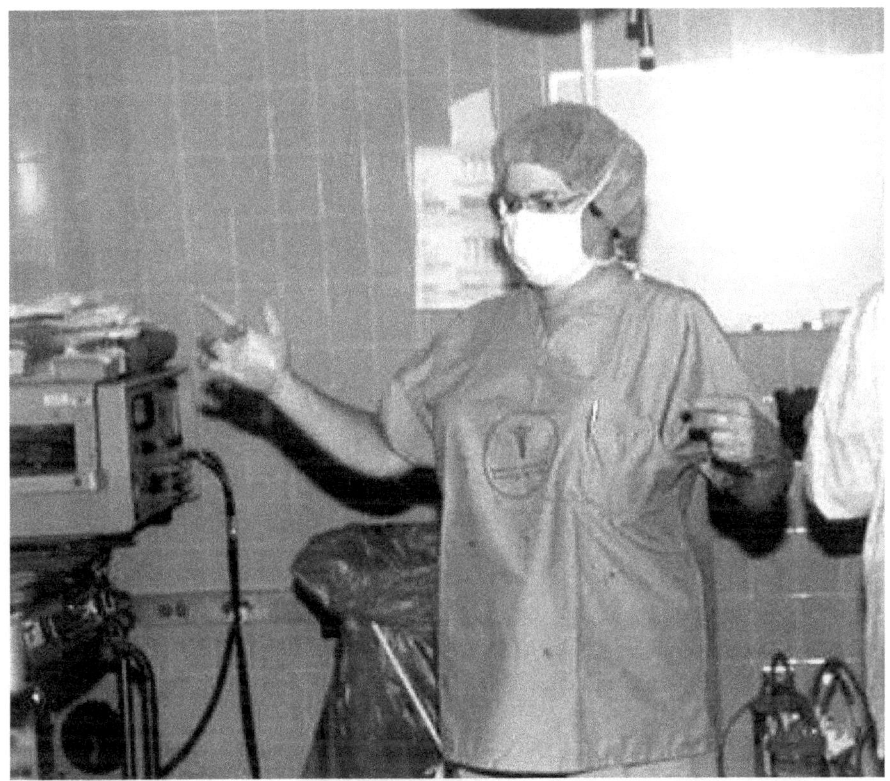

Donna the surgeon

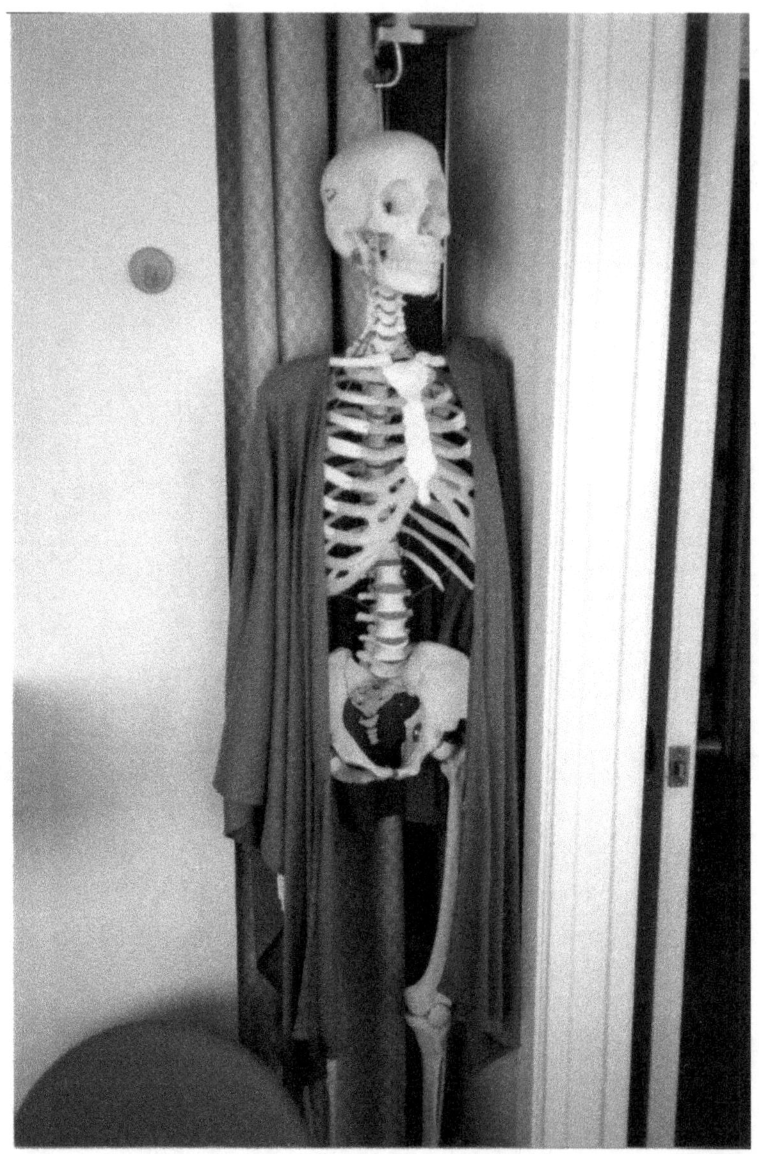

Dolly the skeleton wearing one of the warm ruannas wraps

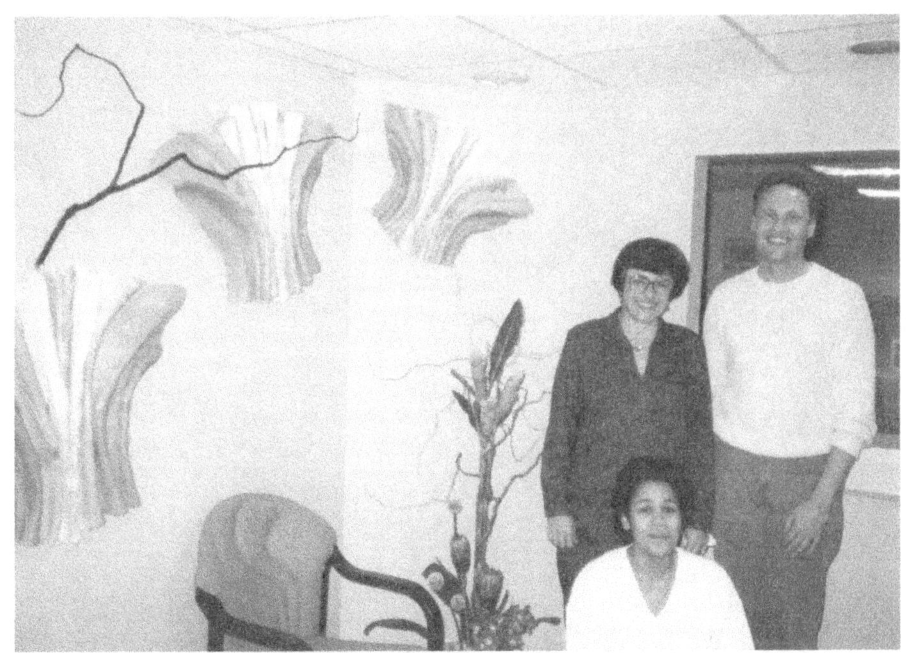

Donna and staff in their new office,

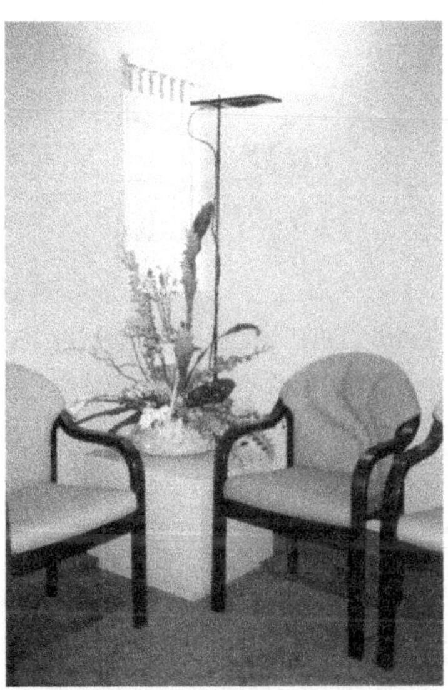

With real art and fresh flowers!

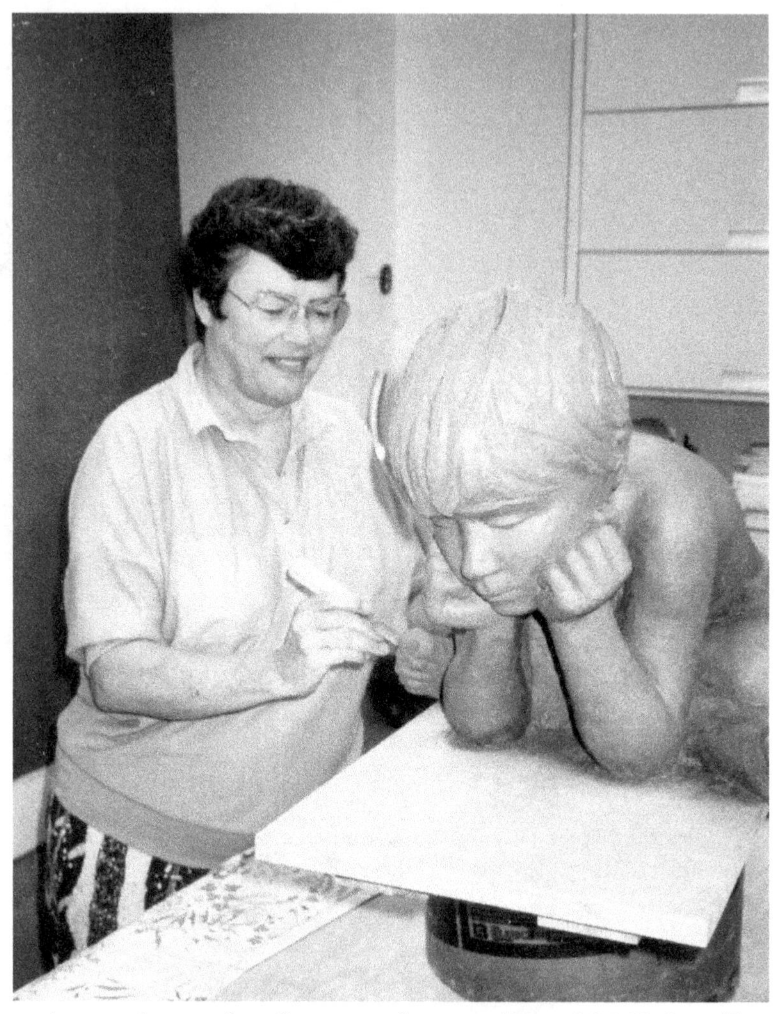

At work on the first sculpture "David Michael"

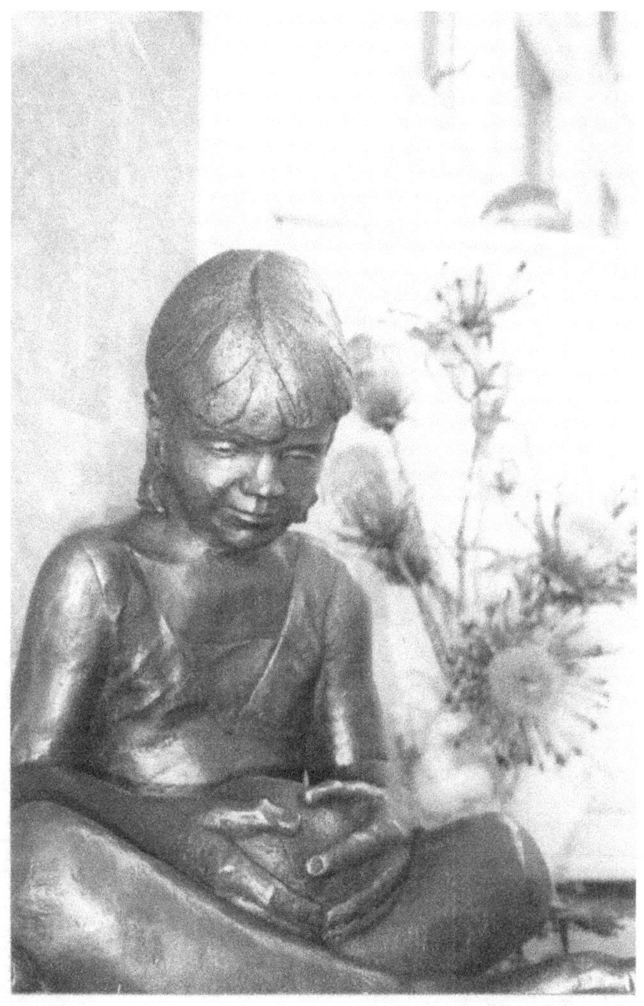

Ariel, whose mother became a physician after getting to know Donna

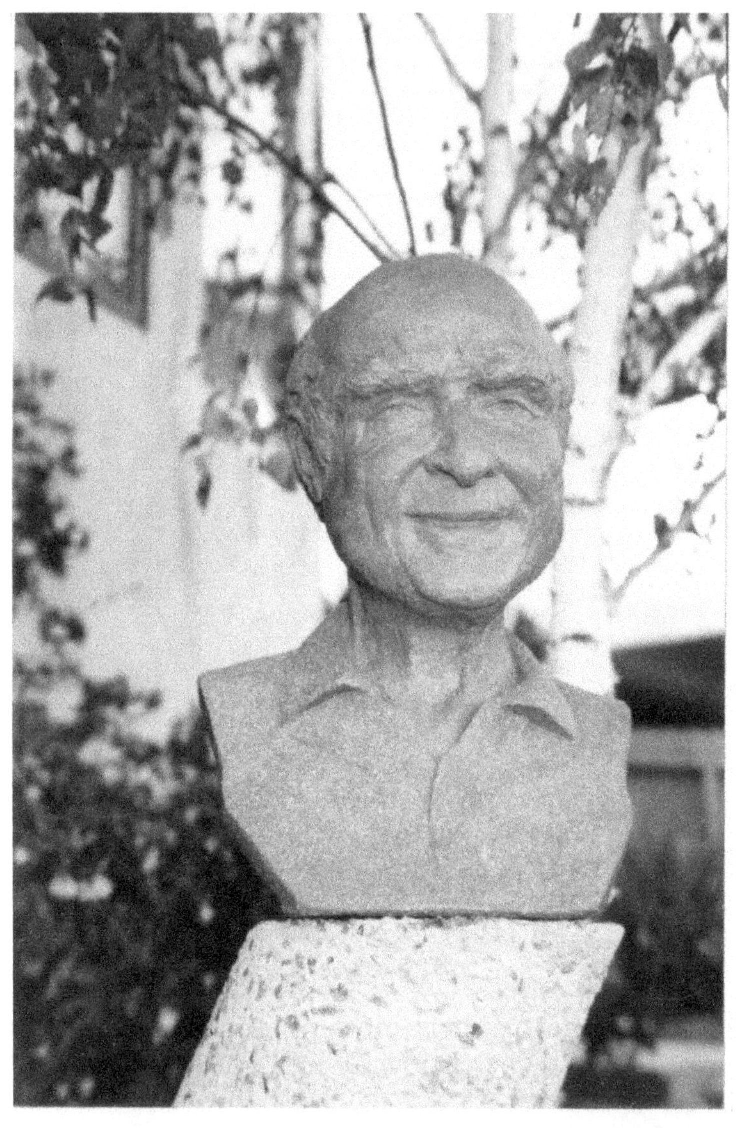

Donna captured nuances of expression

Bust of Erv Polster

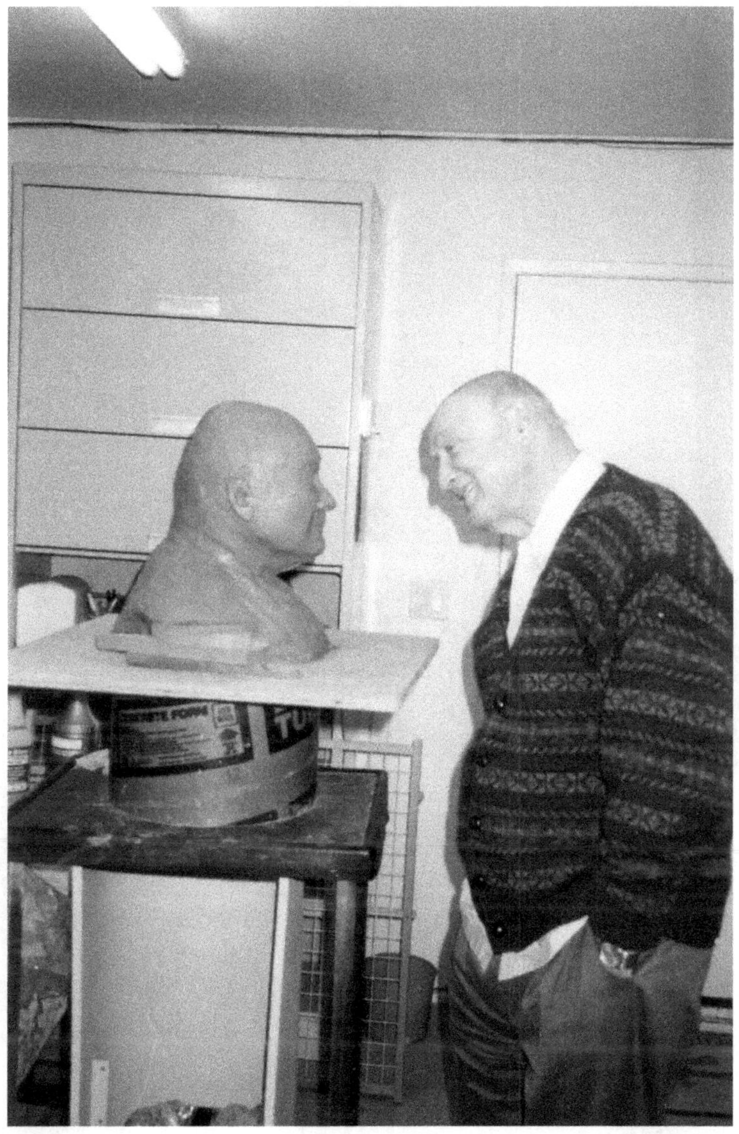

Dimitri admiring the accuracy of his own likeness

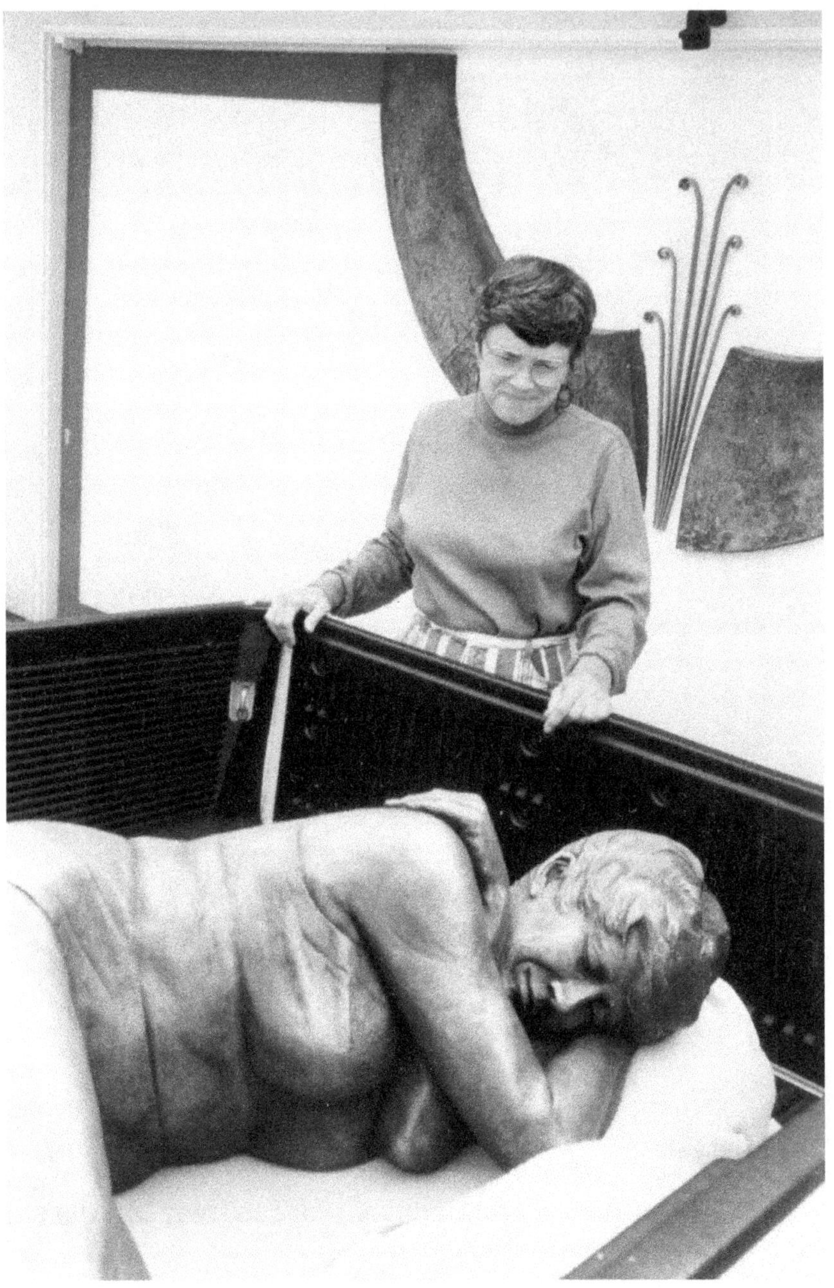

“La Siesta” is delivered after casting

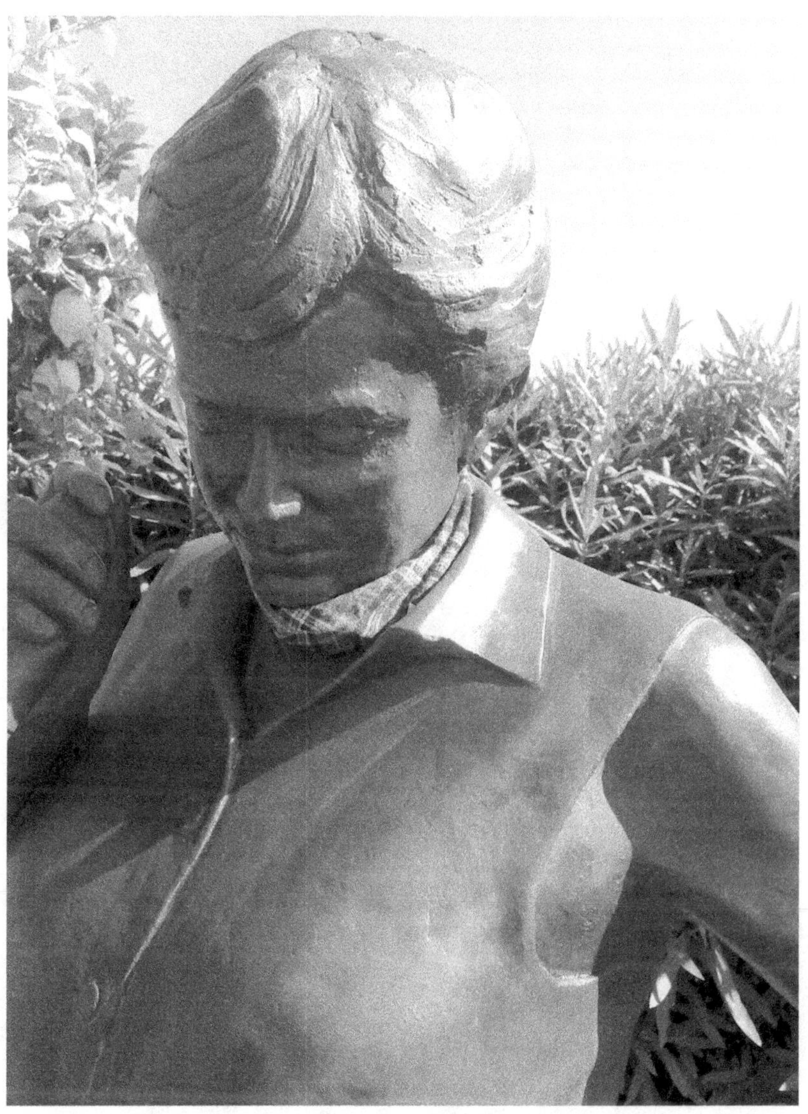

Detail of the self-portrait

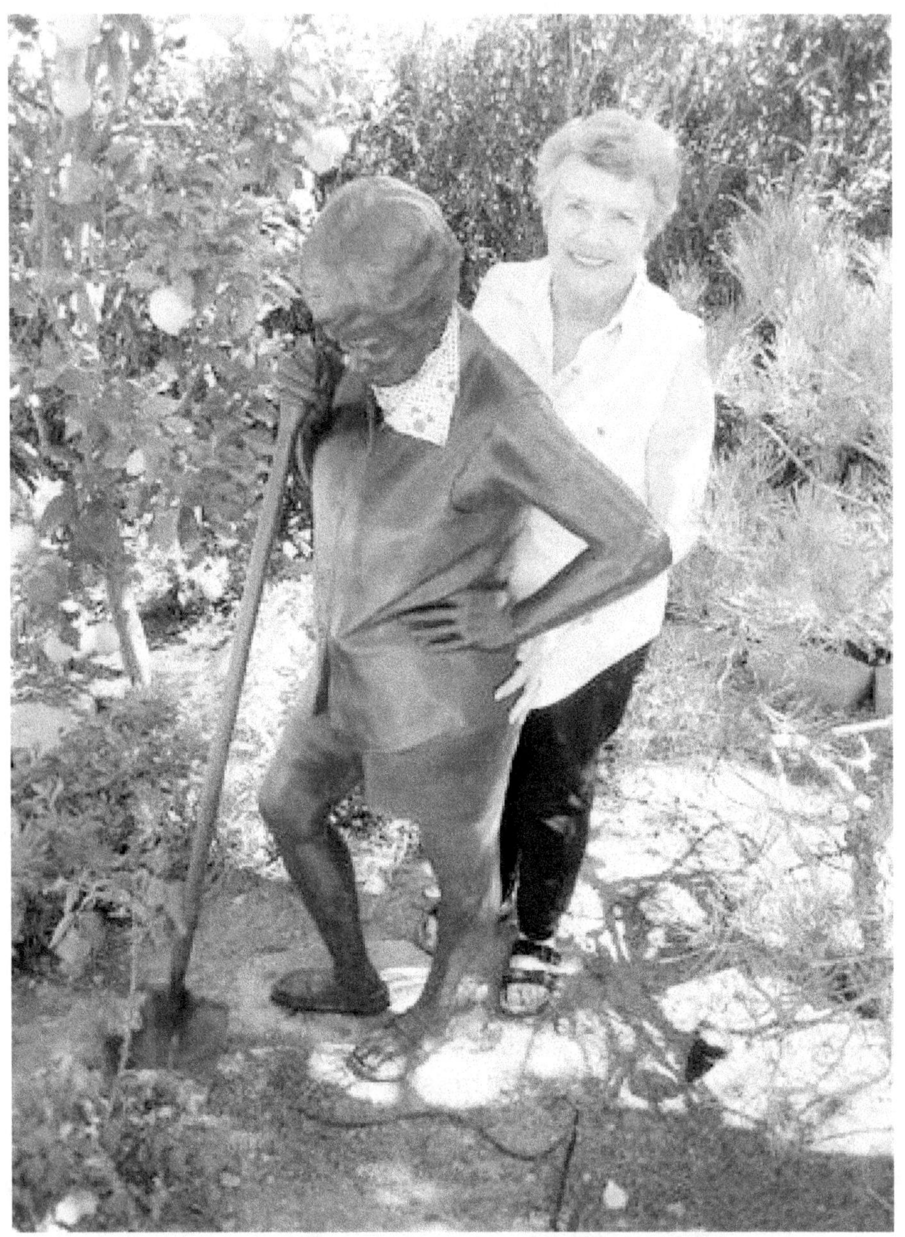

Donna with her self-portrait

Epilogue
The Sacred Trust

> *"Life is not easy for any of us. But what of that? We must have perseverance and above all confidence in ourselves. We must believe that we are gifted for something and that this thing must be attained."*
>
> — Marie Curie, chemist and physicist

Milo Brooks came of age as the profession of medicine itself came of age. The Flexner Report of 1910, commissioned by the AMA and the Carnegie Foundation, called for the closing of small medical schools, the introduction of science and evidence-based teaching, the raising of standards for admission, and the control of clinical instruction in hospitals to be given to medical schools. Flexner's views on the profession still dominate today. While Milo benefitted greatly from his location, where it was not only possible but likely that an eminent professor could personally come to know each of his students as a human being, he also benefitted from his homestead and community.

Perseverance, a confident sense of purpose, adaptability and imagination saturated his world, and his character. Working his way through the years it took to become a doctor, Milo did not abandon his goal except for ways to earn enough to save for the next tuition bill. He became an accomplished teacher out of this necessity, and was dedicated to teaching students, colleagues, parents and neighbors for the rest of his life.

In taking on the issues facing a limb deficient child, Milo was the pioneer: creating a team to address all the needs of the family, introducing a multi-disciplinary approach in the clinical setting, and stressing above all that the doctor's role was to model love and respect for the potential of the child. Like most children of the homestead, Milo believed people were capable of great things, no matter what their circumstances. He knew his older brother Maurice could steer the breaking plow, or manage to get his sisters safely home in a blizzard, or bring the team across a prairie fire— and yet Maurice was a child too. He could see his mother avidly engaged in transformation; whether it was to create a literate and educated family without resources, or save enough money from her meager egg sales to assure herself that Milo could continue in school. Milo could not have imagined that he would hold three professorships and found an institute, but he could imagine himself as a healer and knew he must make a real difference, a positive difference, in the lives of those around him.

Similarly, Donna did not know, as she set off to Pomona College to become a physical education teacher, that she would one day be viewed as 'the best' gynecologist and gynecologic surgeon in San Diego. But she did know that whatever path she took, she would give it her best effort. She too became a pioneer in women's medical care, emphasizing prevention, education and the engagement of her patients in their own recovery and eventual flourishing. She exemplified what she wanted medicine to be as a profession, and she adapted her skills but not her standards to the changing demands upon her.

However, Donna sees beyond the grief of her students and colleagues about the state of medical practice today. She now imagines a medicine of the future which is able to use the panoply of technical and informative tools to focus on prevention, to manage chronic disease in ways that encourage and support rather than emphasize medical encounters, and which returns the physician's role to that of a trusted educator whose purpose is improving public health, not merely doing repeated interventions.

The Real Women Project depended upon Donna's knowledge of women's health, on her understanding of the impact of sculpted figures because of her own accomplishment as a sculptor, and on her commitment to education and prevention. For five years the sculptures toured nine science museums across the country as part of the National Sciences Consortium's exhibit "The Changing Face of Women's Health."

Each person who visited this exhibit was challenged to think of beauty, capacity and our shared reality in a new way. When Dolly the skeleton was pulled out of the closet to teach a patient about her own anatomy, Donna was expanding and deepening her role as a physician. Centering diagnosis and treatment only in the hospital, she reflects, limits the perspective on the patient and on the resources available for healing and for health. This puts an artificial institutional boundary on the physician's role. If some aspect of her chronic disease requires that she spend time at a clinic or in a hospital today, Donna is likely to return home with a new insight into what can change.

Recently one of her specialists complained that young residents and physicians do not know the natural course of a given disease or ailment but they only know the momentary snapshot of what confronts them. Donna thinks of reintroducing the hands-on physical examination and history, but instead of Milo's mirror that enabled him to watch how he was handling an infant and the parents' reactions, Donna would film the encounter so that the preceptor and student would be able to watch and correct what was done and what was said. Then, she would buddy medical students and patients within a primary care practice, so that the medical student not only learns the course of the disease, but learns the conditions of health and healing as the patient lives and works.

While some skills, like thosc of surgery, must be taught within the hospital, much of the education around health and prevention can take place wherever the patient has access to the information, or wherever a network of trust and support exists. Experiments across the country are taking place in congregations, in advocacy organizations and with online efforts to make appropriate education readily accessible.

Nothing can replace the impact of a trusted relationship between a true healer and her patient. Donna's experiences since retirement have expanded and transformed her view of how to reach individuals with significant education. In the instances where there is little trust, or no reliable empathetic relationship, Donna sees that animals can bridge the gap. Cathy has worked tirelessly to create programs relying on animals as transitional objects for children and veterans. When one of the thousands of respondents raises a clinical issue, Donna adds her expertise.

It is an essential aspect of the pioneering tradition to learn continually and to seek new opportunities to apply that learning. Milo and Eva went to Mexico to study Spanish; Donna has become adept at using available computer tools to communicate and to learn. Perhaps one of the significant ways future doctors can learn to see patients and persons is in listening to their stories. While time in the clinical setting may be increasingly constrained, the archiving of narratives using information technology makes them available when the student physician is ready for them.

Necessity imposed constant challenges on the pioneers; Milo and his siblings had to be ready to pay attention and to attempt solutions to critical problems at any time. Older brother Maurice had never experienced a prairie fire before he had to save the team of horses in the face of such a blaze. Similarly, Milo practiced medicine in a time of constant innovations, learning to administer new vaccines, new antibiotics, and therapeutic techniques as they came available. During Donna's years in practice both diagnostic tools and surgical techniques changed considerably, and she was frequently the teacher of these innovations to her colleagues.

What creates this constant readiness to learn?

Donna believes no physician ever knows enough, there is no end point to what can be discovered about people and what might help them live healthier lives. However, she knows that the clinical judgment that she exercised was honed both by her experience and by her curiosity. When she speaks of the mystery of the human body, Donna is reverent, as well as intensely driven to know and learn more. Milo and Donna portray in their lives as in their practice lives dedicated both to science and to service. Our pioneer ancestors were scientists: driven by curiosity, constantly experimenting and observing new results, incessantly trying to find replicable methods and replicable results through the skills available to them.

We should not forget, however, that they became pioneers because of imagination. The descendents of Goodwife Brooks in New England undertook the migration and struggles in Iowa and North Dakota because of an imagined world. The innovators who have so changed medicine, from Madame Curie to Jonas Salk to James Watson and Francis Crick, saw beyond what they already knew to something they imagined might be possible. Milo saw beyond the deficits of a limb deficient child's life to what might be achieved if the child were enabled to flourish. Donna saw beyond distress, disease and fear to what might be gained through education, through her skills, and through the transformations wrought by trust and respect between patient and physician. She imagined that the goal was not the end of the encounter with the patient or the completion of surgery, the goal was a more vital woman, engaged in her own care and healing.

Nowhere is this courageous imagination more important than in pain management. Donna struggles daily with the pains associated with her condition, and with the drugs which are given to assist her. Milo cautioned his students not to say that a procedure would not hurt, but rather to show that it was over quickly or could be ignored when something more interesting, like Bosco the hand puppet, engaged the child's attention. We cannot really comprehend the pains that Milo suffered over the loss of his sons Richard and Ron, yet we know from his memoirs that he imagined and kept faith in his ability to help others. This did not remove or eradicate his pain, but certainly it gave him another way to focus his attention.

> *"People are like stained-glass windows. They sparkle and shine when the sun is out, but when the darkness sets in, their true beauty is revealed only if there is a light from within."*
>
> — Elizabeth Kübler-Ross

To all who know her, Donna radiates this light from within, enlightening as well as brightening the lives around her. Perhaps hardest for her is accepting the limitations on what she can and cannot do. She is like the new physicians today: she expects to be able to help in all circumstances, but external constraints not of her choosing require that she redefine her actions. This process of constraint and redefinition is continuous, as in current medical practice. One day may be better than another; one gesture which used to be safe is now painful and puts her at risk.

A young physician today may find that the therapy she expected to use on behalf of her patients has now been circumscribed by insurance policy. One procedure or therapy that the physician learned is effective and safe may no longer be reimbursed, and she may be unable to recommend it to her patient. This is a constant ebb and flow of transformation, and for Donna the patient, it is a reflection of what made her a great physician. No learning is wasted, no adaptation ignored.

As a physician Donna used education to overcome the fears her patients expressed, and she used her wise and attentive listening to hear what they did not say. While she as patient does fear increasing loss of function, Donna as physical therapist knows that managing pain requires management of change. Maintaining a focus on what is possible rather than on the fear of what may be, or guilt about having to ask for help, is the way to sustain her vitality.

Medicine cannot be helpful unless the physician knows the social, environmental, emotional and spiritual aspects of the patient's life. We have seen many medical interventions fail because too little attention has been given to the context of the person's distress. A physician might prescribe home-based oxygen therapy for a patient with respiratory distress, but the patient may be unable to access the oxygen because her income does not expand to cover the additional expense of the increased electricity use, plus the oxygen, or because a care-giver in the family smokes, or because her self-image refuses to let her wear the tubing. Another physician may prescribe a special diet for someone with brittle diabetes, but that person is cooking for growing, athletic sons, and so cooks for her sons rather than for her own needs, and cannot imagine how to do both. Another therapist prescribes increased exercise for a person suffering from low back pain, but that person feels activity increases pain and so avoids exercise and cannot imagine a time when he might be able to add more. The therapist labels the patient noncompliant and does not understand the fears and expectations that limit the person from undertaking the prescribed regimen.

Donna and Milo practiced medicine in the same way that the homesteaders built this country: By doing the task immediately in front of them with full attention, determined to learn how to do the task better. This capacity to focus attention on the specific and immediate need, while sustaining a sense of purpose transcending that need, appears to be a matter of character rather than a professional skill. When the larger sense of purpose is driven both by service and by generosity, all of us are inspired. What new models of medical education would engage and inspire future medical students?

Reflective of the positive impacts technology can have on certain interventions two kinds of medical care are especially successful in 2013, they are trauma care, and rehabilitative care. Both of these areas of medicine are practiced in a team: the nurse, the physical therapist, the social worker, and physicians from many different specialties work together for the best possible outcomes for the patient. Milo Brooks said to Donna that it was critical that she be liked by the nurses. He put together multi-disciplinary teams to address the needs of the limb deficient child and the family. When he first began dealing with pediatric prosthetics, his first stop was at the engineering department. The comprehensive skills that such a team offers transcend specialty care, and provide the diverse resources of support that patients need to heal and recover after traumatic injury or after an intervention that requires rehabilitation.

The ways of working in a team have not traditionally been taught in medical school, and it has been left to the temperament of the physician to determine whether such teamwork worked. Donna cultivated her team, nurtured them over several years, and knew that the care they could deliver together was greater than the care any one of them could give alone. As information technology eliminates the need for the emphasis on rote learning of data, medical students educated in multi-disciplinary teams will be better able to cultivate the clinical judgment regarding allocations of skills and resources for the patient's benefit.

As efforts are made to change reimbursement from the fee-for-service model with its accompanying side-effects of unnecessary and wasteful interventions as well as false expectations on the part of patients, medical students can learn--as Milo and Donna knew--that the practice of medicine is not about financial reward. One of the great sources of waste, both in dollars and in the time of physicians, is the fact that over half of the prescriptions given are either never filled or if filled never taken as instructed. In addition to never filling a prescription, a high percentage of patients with chronic illnesses skip doses or cut medication is half in order to reduce the need for refilling the prescription.

The common reason given is that medicine costs more than the patient can afford, but the underlying reason is the lack of understanding of the need for or benefits of the medication. This is primarily an aspect of education, rather than an issue of willful 'noncompliance'. As physicians are educated to work in a team, and to understand the ecology of care in addition to the episode of care, they can better fulfill their role as educators. Both Milo and Donna were responsible for the continuum of care: they did not hand their patients off to another practitioner during the course of an illness or treatment, and they did not see their patients only in acute need.

Another of the arguments made in reform efforts is that there is a significant shortage of primary care physicians because the American model is both specialty care and hospital-based. Many of the innovative models being tried involve the use of non-physicians to deliver primary care under the supervision of a physician, thus expanding the reach of the physician's skills, while at the same time overcoming the gaps caused by a focus on specialty care. In Milo's practice, he held well-baby and immunization clinics as fundamental to his ability to care for his patients. Donna enjoyed obstetrics because it enabled her to see healthy as well as sick individuals. Both Milo and Donna used their primary care platform for the education of patients in healthy choices, and took the time to be sure that those messages were understood. This change of focus would further expand the public health model of care away from our current disease-care model. It would recover the practical intelligence and common sense of seeking to do only what is effective, while not taking action when such action would make no difference.

Barbara Levy, Donna's student, fears that medicine is becoming a trade rather than a profession, in part because physicians now seek rewards and recognition (in terms of hours, compensation and limitation on responsibility) rather than constantly improving performance. Donna knows that the interactions that she and Barbara shared, from Barbara's first year as a medical student, helped to show what was involved in dedication to patient care and to excellence in the profession.

Over several years of apprenticeship or mentoring, a medical student can see not only the natural course of illness, the consequences of treatment, and the personhood of the patient, but can see how a physician learns, how the art of empathy is applied, how colleagues can and must cooperate. Idealistic students with such mentorship are not forced over the burdened years of medical education into a cynical battle with time, but can aspire to become practitioners constantly seeking excellence, constantly curious about new knowledge and skills, and constantly affirming their service. Barbara worries that there are too few mentors available.

One of the themes in the Brooks family traditions is the emphasis on common sense and practical solutions. Often in medical interactions the language used creates barriers rather than communicates. For instance, the word 'dementia' as a label is dangerous because not only of the legal and social implications that the person so labeled is incompetent, but because many people will avoid discussions of real issues due to their fears of the word. Cognitive loss is a far more accurate term, without the baggage of negativity associated with dementia. Pain is another such word, where we have subjective interpretations of meaning which can compromise the medical care and the understanding of what is needed. Milo first encountered this problem when he recorded that a baker described his condition in terms of his work, but the resident taking the history did not understand that language and came to erroneous conclusions. Donna has always been particularly careful about the language she uses as part of her sense of obligation to connect with others and which she does with practical accuracy. We need to remind medical students that their language must be a tool for communication, not an isolating jargon, or a barrier causing fear or withdrawal.

Sometimes we may grieve the pace of our own lives, or the loss of what we see as a less fraught life for our ancestors. No one could claim that EE Brooks, Melvina and their children lived lives of less demanding struggle than those we live in 2013. The pioneer struggles were clear, the need for mutual cooperation a matter of survival, and the moral obligation to help others meant that life was lived with a focus on action. Perhaps it is that clarity which is missing as we attempt to juggle the complex priorities of current life.

One of the lessons of the homesteading life made evident throughout the Brooks family history is that although imagination and faith in a greater purpose were fundamental to all that they knew, action was directed toward immediate needs, not toward an ambition. Milo took the variety of jobs to pay his tuition and to survive, even though when he reflected upon these demands he knew that eventually he would be a better physician if he was able to understand the diversity of his patients' lives. Yet beyond the emphasis on this practical intelligence, we see in the pioneer heritage a cultivation of the skills of acute observation and adaptability. We look in awe at their efforts and their courage, and may give less notice to their ability to focus astutely on what they needed to learn to do the next task at hand.

Those who did not succeed on the homestead were those who could not adapt their own skills and traditions to the new context or to the constantly changing external conditions of their lives. Melvina's determination that all of her children be educated was no doubt driven by her very practical guidance that people must above all strive to understand each other and the world they shared. Like many women on the homestead, and like Eva Brooks during the busiest years of Milo's practice when her children were young, Melvina looked beyond the hardship to the world of possibility. For the Brooks family and descendents the possibilities were in service through the relationships they made. Their astonishing fidelity to communication with each other is a testament to the value they placed on these relationships. Donna's commitment to acting as an advocate and caring counselor to all who need her continues that tradition.

While both Maurice and Milo consciously sought careers away from the hardships of farming on the prairie, they did not abandon the skills of observation, craftsmanship and contribution to their communities. We see the evolution of adaptation over Donna's life: from physical education to physical therapy to anatomist to obstetrician to gynecologic surgeon to sculptor to patient advocate. The pioneer above all carries on: In the face of blizzards, fire, crop failures and personal tragedy. While Milo pioneered care for limb deficient children, he lived his life with that pioneer endurance. Donna now approaches her eightieth birthday with curiosity and with all the disciplines of continuous learning that made her such an exemplary mentor.

Can we create a medical education which inspires students to see themselves as pioneers, adapting knowledge to new challenges and helping their patients to flourish as they deal with change? The mystery of human beings remains as enticing as when Hippocrates said

> *Wherever the art of medicine is loved,*
> *there also is love of humanity.*

Milo Brooks and Donna Brooks have shown that their true calling as healers was to find ways to show that love. For future physicians, their lives provide a beacon of hope that dedication and service to the art of medicine will always lead to something positive to do.

Major Medical Advances

From Milo's Time to the Present

1900 For every 1000 live births, six to nine women died of pregnancy related complications and approximately 100 infants died before age one year.

1900s British obstetrician James Blundell performs transfusions on women hemorrhaging from post-partum child birth.

1900 Austrian-American Karl Landsteiner describes blood biocompatability and rejection, presents the ABO system.

1908 First successful transfusion using Landsteiner's ABO typing technique.

1910 Flexner report on medical education published

1911 Madame Curie discovers radium.

1912 Polish biochemist Casimir Funk identifies vitamins.

1914 Dr. Paul Dudley White publishes the first study of coagulation of the blood.

1917 British physician Dr. Ivan Magill invents the endotracheal tube.

1920 Scientist/ aviator Charles A. Lindberg first oxygen ation of perfusion fluid driven by compressed oxygen gas.

1922 Insulin first used to treat diabetes.

1923—27 Vaccines for diphtheria, Pertussis, tetanus and tuberculosis developed

1929 Penicillin: the action of this antibiotic was first observed by British bacteriologist Sir Alexander Fleming. Introduced in general medicine post 1945.

1931 First use of phenobarbitone for anesthesia.

1935 First successful application of the heart-lung machine for extracorporeal circulation in an animal (cat).

1937 The first blood bank started using a 2% solution of sodium citrate. Refrigerated blood lasted ten days.

1939 The use of plasma is preferred over whole blood for the treatment of shock, burns and open wounds.

1943 Selman Abraham Waksman discovered the antibiotic streptomycin used in the treatment of tuberculosis and other diseases.

1948 National Heart Institute enacts the Framington (Massachusetts) study to study the effects of factors influencing coronary artery disease.
The project is ongoing.

1951 First kidney transplantation, Peter Bent Brigham Hospital, Boston.

1952 Paul Zoll develops the first cardiac pacemaker.

1953 James Watson and Francis Crick describe the structure of DNA

1955 Jonas Edward Salk's killed-virus vaccine against poliomyelitis declared safe.

1957 Introduction of the use of ultrasound to visualize the heart non-invasively.

1958-1961 Thalidomide used to prevent nausea in pregnancy and withdrawn.

1960 The contraceptive pill is approved by the FDA

1960s Vaccines against hepatitis, mumps, measles, rubella

1960 Medtronic develops the first fully implantable pacemaker.

1967 The first coronary bypass operation using the patient's native saphenous vein as an autograft.

1970 Publication of *Our Bodies, Ourselves* influences women's health care

1975 Introduction of computerized axial tomography, the "CAT-scanner."

1970's First artificial joint replacements take place in the United States

1978 First test tube baby born in the United Kingdom

1980 WHO announces smallpox is eradicated

1981 Toxic shock syndrome identified

1983 HIV the virus is identified

1992 MRI invented

1990 Human Genome Project announced, Declared completed in 2003

1996 Dolly the sheep is the first cloned animal

2007 Introduction of the production of embryonic stem cells from skin cells

The Archive

Photographs from approximately 1870 to the present

Genealogy of the Brooks and Crawford families from 1591 to present

Milo Brooks Memoirs, three different versions with handwritten originals

Memoirs by Maurice Brooks

Correspondence from family members and from patients and colleagues

Back-up documents to the memoirs, such as building plans

Women's Medical College of Pennsylvania history, photographs, interviews

Diplomas and awards for Milo Brooks and Donna Lou Brooks

This is Your Life celebration of Milo Brooks by The Rotary Club

Pamphlets, articles and depositions on the Child Amputee Prosthetics Project

Photographic record of Donna's practice and various surgeries

Photographic studies of Donna's sculptures

Materials of The Real Woman Project and Henry's World

Photographic albums recording Brooks and Crawford family reunions

Newspaper articles on the wedding anniversaries of EE and Melvina Brooks

Obituaries on various Brooks and Crawford family members

The *Brooks Babbler* newsletter from 1935 to 2012

Two volumes of letters of appreciation on Donna's retirement.

Bibliography

Barry, John M., *The Great Influenza; The Story of the Deadliest Pandemic in History*, Penguin, New York, 2005

Biro, David, *One Hundred Days, My Unexpected Journey from Doctor to Patient*, Vintage, New York, 2001

Chesworth, Jennifer, Editor, *The Ecology of Health*, Sage, London, 1996

Ehrenreich, Barbara, and English, Deirdre, *For Her Own Good*, Doubleday, new York, 1978

Gawande, Atul, *The Checklist Manifesto, How to Get Things Right*, Picador, New York, 2010

Grant, Ted and Carter, Sandy, *Women in Medicine: a Celebration of their Work*, Firefly Books, Buffalo, 2004

Halvorson, George C., Isham, George, J., *Epidemic of Care, A Call for Safter, Better, and More Accountable Health Care*, Jossey-Bass, San Francisco, 2003

Leavitt, Judith Walzer and Numbers, Ronald L., Ed., *Sickness and Health in America*, Readings in the History of Medicine and Public Health, Third Edition Revised, The University of Wisconsin Press, Madison, 1997

Malcolm, River, *Essays of a Legacy, Portraits of Women Physicians*, La Jolla, 2000 Donna L. Brooks, M.D.

Moore, Wendy, *The Knife Man*, Doubleday, New York, 2005

Porter, Roy, *The Greatest Benefit to Mankind, A Medical History of Humanity*, W.W. Norton, New York, 1997

Reiser, Stanley Joel, *Technological Medicine, The Changing World of Doctors and Patients*, Cambridge University Press, New York, 2009

Seifter, Julian with Seifter, Betsy, *After the Diagnosis, Transcending Chronic Illness*, Simon and Schuster, New York, 2012

Taylor, Jill Bolte, *My Stroke of Insight, A Brain Scientist's Personal Journey*, Plume, Penguin, New York, 2009

Topol, Eric J., *The Creative Destruction of Medicine, How the Digital Revolution will Create Better Health Care*, Basic Books, New York 2012

HEATHER WOOD ION is a chief executive and cultural anthropologist who specializes in turning around troubled organizations. She has taught in various medical schools and consulted on many aspects of change in healthcare.

Heather Wood's first book, *Third-class Ticket*, has been translated into Italian, Hindi, Japanese, and Chinese, and is currently being made into a feature film.

Another book, with Saul Levine M.D., *Against Terrible Odds*, applies her knowledge of social and cultural recovery to the profound issues of individual resilience.

www.ingramcontent.com/pod-product-compliance
Lightning Source LLC
Chambersburg PA
CBHW061306110426
42742CB00012BA/2076

* 9 7 8 0 9 8 9 8 0 5 6 0 5 *